国家"十一五"重点图书

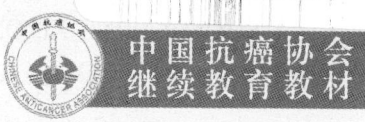

中国肿瘤医师临床实践指南丛书

中枢神经系统常见肿瘤
诊疗纲要

Clinical Practice Guidelines for Central Nervous System Tumors

第 2 版

中国抗癌协会神经肿瘤专业委员会／编著

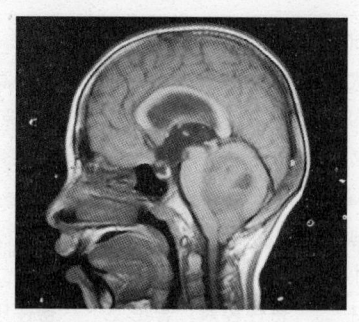

 北京大学医学出版社

ZHONGSHUSHENJING XITONG CHANGJIAN ZHONGLIU
ZHENLIAO GANGYAO

图书在版编目（CIP）数据

中枢神经系统常见肿瘤诊疗纲要 / 中国抗癌协会神经肿瘤专业委员会编著. —北京：北京大学医学出版社，2012.9

ISBN 978-7-5659-0445-5

Ⅰ.①中… Ⅱ.①中… Ⅲ.①中枢神经系统疾病-肿瘤-诊疗 Ⅳ.①R739.4

中国版本图书馆 CIP 数据核字（2012）第 205508 号

中枢神经系统常见肿瘤诊疗纲要（第 2 版）

编　　著：中国抗癌协会神经肿瘤专业委员会
出版发行：北京大学医学出版社（电话：010-82802230）
地　　址：(100191) 北京市海淀区学院路 38 号 北京大学医学部院内
网　　址：http://www.pumpress.com.cn
E - mail：booksale@bjmu.edu.cn
印　　刷：北京画中画印刷有限公司
经　　销：新华书店
责任编辑：苗　旺　　责任校对：金彤文　　责任印制：张京生
开　　本：889mm×1194mm 1/32　印张：3　字数：76 千字
版　　次：2012 年 9 月第 2 版　2012 年 9 月第 1 次印刷
书　　号：ISBN 978-7-5659-0445-5
定　　价：12.50 元
版权所有，违者必究
（凡属质量问题请与本社发行部联系退换）

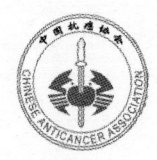

中国肿瘤医师临床实践指南丛书编委会

主　　编　徐光炜　郝希山

编委会成员　（按姓氏笔画排序）

于世英	万德森	马　军	王耀平
方伟岗	方志沂	叶胜龙	朴炳奎
朱正纲	朱雄增	任　军	刘淑俊
孙建衡	李春海	杨仁杰	杨秉辉
吴一龙	吴沛宏	冈华庆	沈镇宙
张汝刚	张宗卫	陆道培	陈忠平
邵志敏	郑　树	施诚仁	洪明晃
倪泉兴	徐万鹏	高宗人	曹雪涛
董志伟	蒋国梁	韩德民	储大同
管忠震			

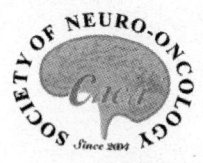

编者名单

编著/中国抗癌协会神经肿瘤专业委员会

组长　陈忠平　中山大学肿瘤防治中心神经外科/神经肿瘤科
组员　（按姓氏拼音排序）
　　　卞修武　第三军医大学西南医院病理研究所
　　　胡超苏　上海市复旦大学附属肿瘤医院放疗科
　　　兰　青　苏州大学第二附属医院神经外科
　　　李文良　天津医科大学附属肿瘤医院神经外科
　　　梁碧玲　中山大学第二附属医院影像科
　　　孙晓非　中山大学肿瘤防治中心化疗内科
　　　王贵怀　首都医科大学附属北京天坛医院神经外科
　　　夏云飞　中山大学肿瘤防治中心放疗科
　　　肖建平　中国医学科学院肿瘤医院放疗科
　　　杨学军　天津医科大学总医院神经外科
　　　游　潮　四川大学华西医院神经外科
　　　于春江　北京三博脑科医院神经外科
　　　于士柱　天津医科大学总医院神经病理科
　　　章　翔　第四军医大学西京医院全军神经外科研究所
　　　张俊平　北京三博脑科医院神经肿瘤化疗科
　　　赵世光　哈尔滨医科大学第一临床医学院神经外科
　　　朱剑虹　复旦大学附属华山医院神经外科

编辑秘书　杨群英　赛　克　刘巧丹

序　言

进入21世纪后，癌症的死亡率已跃居国内各种死因之首，尤其以40～65岁的中年组为甚，究其原因，恐与人口老龄化、吸烟恶习、工业化的进程及城市化的发展有关。世界上发达的工业化国家其癌症年发病率超过300/10万，其因盖出于此。据世界卫生组织统计，发展中国家的癌症发病率仅为150/10万，但随着经济的发展，癌症发病率也将会相应地增长。我国癌症的发病，近年恐已近200/10万，而上海市则已达300/10万水平。传统的生活贫困地区的常见肿瘤如食管癌、胃癌、肝癌等的发病率仍居高不下，而富裕国家的肺癌、乳腺癌、结肠癌等多发肿瘤却已快速增长，大有后来居上之势，致使我国的肿瘤防治面临两方面的压力，今后二三十年内癌症的发病及死亡恐有增无减，前途颇为堪忧。

当然，控制癌症的策略重在预防，应坚持不懈地贯彻预防为主之原则。但在现实生活中，每日需要处理的是大量现患的癌症患者。鉴于癌症的防治研究近年来取得快速的发展，对癌症本质的认识逐渐加深，新的诊断技术及治疗方法也层出不穷，知识更新甚快，颇有紧于追赶的日新月异之感；再则我国幅地广阔，人口众多，各地区间、不同医院间差别颇大，由于对疾病的认知不一，诊治方法又各有不同，导致治疗效果也就有较大差距。

因此加强癌症防治知识的继续教育，规范各种癌症的诊治方法实乃当务之急。国外虽有NCCN等各种指南，但因国情不同，人种有异，而仅可供参考。有鉴于此，经多次酝酿，决定由中国抗癌协会组织出版系列性的以各种常见癌症的诊疗方法为主的继续教育教材,以提高专业及非专业临床医师对各相关专业领域的基本知识和诊疗水平,计划每4～5年再版一次以更新其内容。与此相对应的还将同时出版各种癌症的诊疗指南,具体地规范各种癌症的诊疗工作,主要介绍适应我国国情的诊疗方案,也将介绍国外的新进展及国内经济欠发达地区应努力做到的最基本要求。考虑到诊疗工作知识更新的快速,此指南将1～2年再版一次,以适应临床工作之需。

由于此一系列性专业书籍分别由各专业委员会集中国内从事该方面工作的著名专家分工负责撰写,因此专业水平应属一流,但鉴于各种癌症及主题各有不同,文风也各异,更由于初次组织如此众多的专家撰写,错误、不足或考虑不周之处在所难免,盼读者诸君能予以谅解,并欢迎批评指正,以便再版时能有所改进。盼本系列读物之问世,将有助于提高我国癌症的诊疗水平。

徐光炜
中国抗癌协会第4、5届理事长
2007年3月26日

前　言

原发性脑肿瘤是十大常见致死肿瘤之一。根据美国资料，与肿瘤相关的死亡原因中，脑肿瘤在20～39岁男性系第1位，女性为第5位。胶质细胞瘤是中枢神经系统（central nervous system, CNS）最常见的原发性肿瘤，其临床预后相差甚远，虽然一些低级别胶质细胞瘤可以治愈，但多数胶质细胞瘤，特别是高级别胶质细胞瘤患者预后不佳。而一些高度恶性的CNS肿瘤，如原发性中枢神经系统淋巴瘤、原发性中枢神经系统生殖细胞瘤，通过合理的治疗，疗效颇好，甚至可以达到治愈。脑转移瘤是颅内最常见的恶性病变，发生率远超过原发恶性脑肿瘤。在全身恶性肿瘤中约有20%～40%的患者会出现脑转移，这些晚期肿瘤患者通过积极的治疗，也能获得延长生存时间、提高生存质量的效果。然而，要达到良好的临床治疗结果，特别是恶性脑肿瘤，多学科合作的综合治疗是前提，而规范化治疗则是基本保障。为此，中国抗癌协会神经肿瘤专业委员会配合中国抗癌协会系列参考丛书——《神经系统肿瘤》，参考欧美发达国家的临床指引，结合中国特点，对中枢神经系统常见（恶性）肿瘤制定相应的诊疗纲要（2010年第1版），供神经肿瘤相关临床工作者参考，对规范治疗和提高我国神经系统肿瘤的治疗效果起到了积极的作用。本次再版是在2010年版基础上做了一些修改和补充，内容包括主要的神经系统常见肿瘤：星形细胞瘤、室管膜瘤、髓母细胞瘤、原发性中枢神经系统淋巴瘤、原发性中枢神经系统生殖细胞肿瘤和脑转移瘤。

陈忠平
中国抗癌协会神经肿瘤专业委员会主任委员
2012年7月

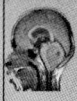

目 录

第一章　高级别胶质细胞肿瘤 …………… 1

第二章　低级别浸润性胶质细胞瘤 ………… 9

第三章　室管膜瘤和间变性室管膜瘤………… 15

第四章　髓母细胞瘤/中枢神经系统原始神经

外胚层肿瘤……………………… 23

第五章　原发性中枢神经系统淋巴瘤………… 31

第六章　原发性中枢神经系统生殖细胞肿瘤

………………………………… 37

第七章　脑转移瘤 ……………………… 43

第八章　神经系统肿瘤常用化疗方案………… 51

第九章　神经系统肿瘤常用放疗方案………… 55

附录一　纲要参考的循证医学依据级别 …… 61

附录二　英文缩略语表 ………………… 63

附录三　参考文献 ……………………… 65

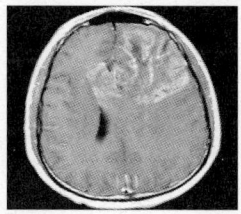

第一章
高级别胶质细胞肿瘤

高级别胶质细胞肿瘤

高级别胶质细胞肿瘤主要是间变性星形细胞瘤（anaplastic astrocytoma，AA）、间变性少突胶质细胞瘤（anaplastic oligodendroglioma，AO）、间变性少突-星形细胞瘤（anaplastic oligodendro-astrocytoma，AOA）（WHO Ⅲ级）及胶质母细胞瘤（glioblastoma，GBM）（WHO Ⅳ级），是成人中最常见的原发性脑肿瘤。GBM占所有胶质细胞瘤半数以上，发病高峰年龄为45～55岁。高级别侵袭性星形细胞肿瘤常弥漫浸润至周围组织，甚至穿过中线侵犯对侧脑组织。

临床表现包括颅内压增高症状、癫痫发作、神经系统定位症状以及瘤周水肿相关症状等。在影像学上，常表现为大范围水肿及肿块占位效应，MRI增强后可见明显强化。而且在肿瘤周围水肿区可有肿瘤细胞，因此这个区域常被认定为肿瘤靶区。

影响患者预后的重要因素有组织学类型、年龄、KPS（Karnofsky Performance Scale）、症状类型及持续时间和手术切除范围等。

治疗应是包括手术、放疗、化疗等方法的综合手段。手术的目的是在保护神经功能的前提下最大范围地切除肿瘤，获取病理诊断，减轻颅内高压及局部压迫所引起的症状，利于放疗、化疗等辅助治疗手段的实施。研究显示，在高级别胶质细胞肿瘤中，肿瘤切除超过98%的患者有明显的生存获益。

不管是在全切除术后还是活检术后，高级别胶质细胞瘤都需要行术后放射治疗，常规分割外照射放疗是高级别胶质细胞瘤的标准治疗。推荐放疗剂量为54～60Gy（1.8～2Gy/次）。

对于老年患者可考虑适当缩短疗程。治疗区域应包括瘤床及周围水肿带外放 2～3cm 区域，或对比增强的肿瘤体积外放 2.5cm 边界。

对高级别胶质细胞瘤，化疗有助于提高患者的无进展生存时间及平均生存时间。近年的研究提示，化疗与放疗联合使用治疗高级别胶质细胞瘤，能提高患者中位生存期。术后同期放疗联合化疗，对提高 GBM 患者生存率有益。目前化疗用药/方案主要有替莫唑胺、亚硝脲类（如 BCNU、ACNU 等）、铂类、鬼臼毒素类（如 VM-26）及 PCV 方案等。新的分子靶向药物如贝伐单抗（bevacizumab），是一种抗血管生成药物，2009 年美国食品及药物管理局（FDA）批准其用于治疗复发 GBM，可以单用，也可联合 CPT-11、BCNU、替莫唑胺化疗。贝伐单抗单用或联合化疗药物对间变性胶质细胞瘤也有效。但贝伐单抗可导致潜在严重不良反应，如影响伤口愈合、引起高血压、肠穿孔和血栓栓塞等。

间变性胶质细胞瘤[a]/胶质母细胞瘤

诊疗流程

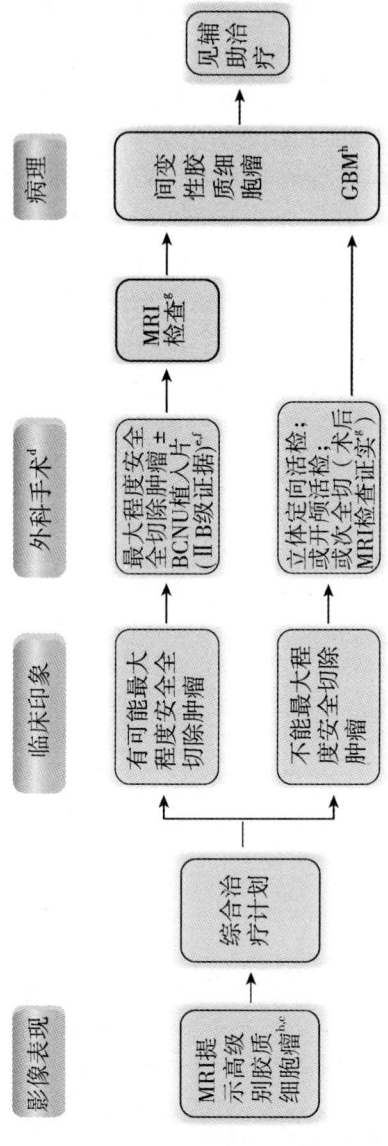

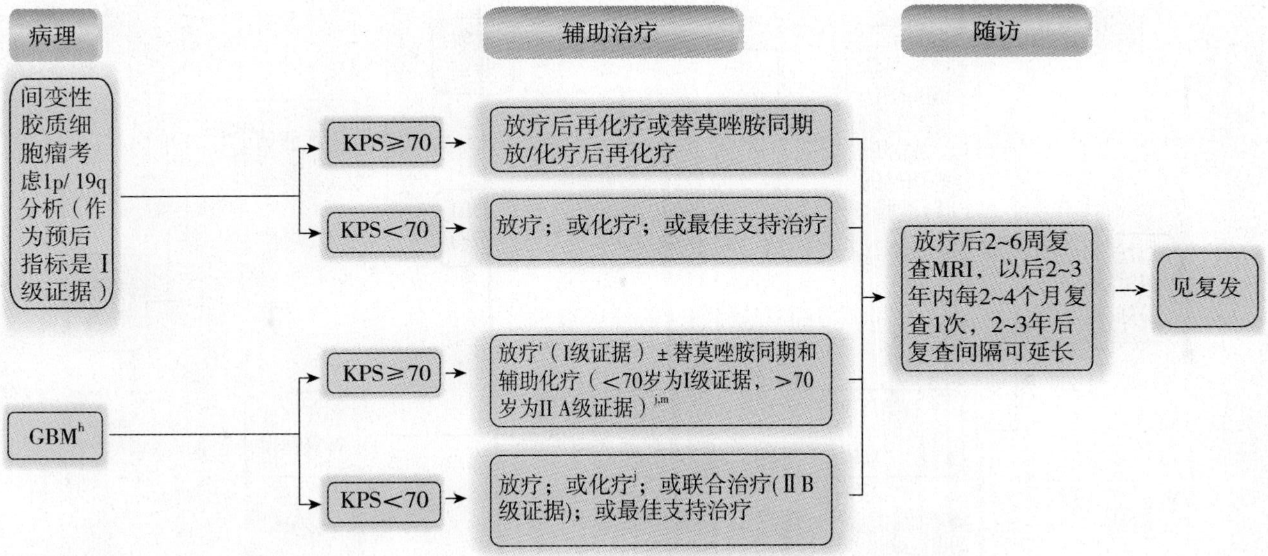

第一章 高级别胶质细胞肿瘤

病理

- 间变性胶质细胞瘤考虑1p/19q分析（作为预后指标是I级证据）
  - KPS≥70 → 放疗后再化疗或替莫唑胺同期放化疗后再化疗
  - KPS<70 → 放疗；或化疗；或最佳支持治疗

- GBM[h]
  - KPS≥70 → 放疗（I级证据）±替莫唑胺同期和辅助化疗（<70岁为I级A级证据，>70岁为II A级证据）[i,j,m]
  - KPS<70 → 放疗；或化疗；或联合治疗（II B级证据）；或最佳支持治疗

辅助治疗

随访

放疗后2~6周复查MRI，以后每2~4个月复查1次，2~3年后复查间隔可延长 → 见复发

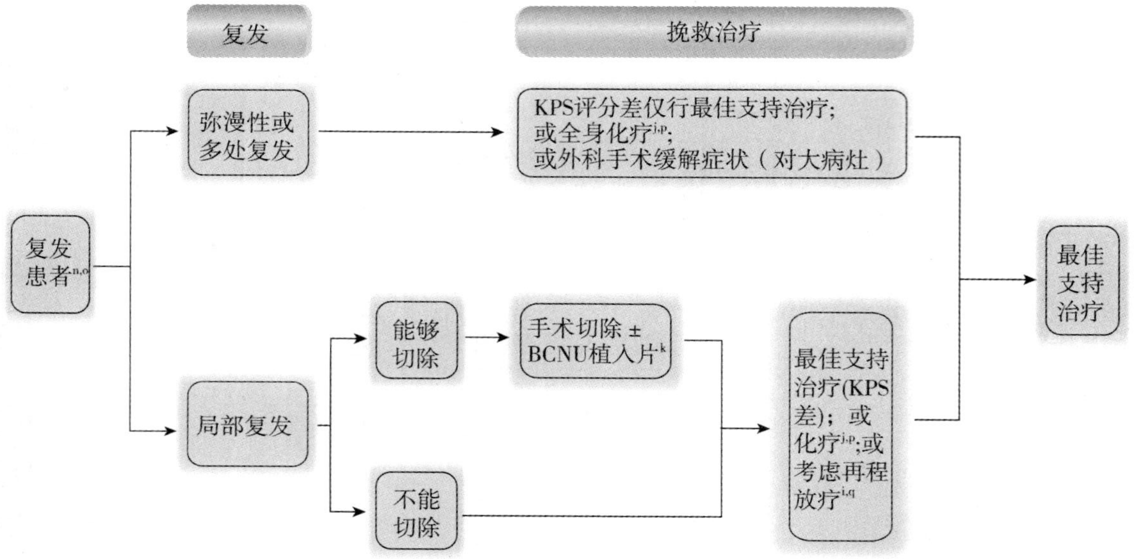

中枢神经系统常见肿瘤诊疗纲要

复发

复发患者[n,o] → 弥漫性或多处复发 → **挽救治疗** → KPS评分差仅行最佳支持治疗[p]；或全身化疗[j]；或外科手术缓解症状（对大病灶）→ 最佳支持治疗

复发患者[n,o] → 局部复发 → 能够切除 → 手术切除±BCNU植入片[k] → 最佳支持治疗（KPS差；化疗[j]；或考虑再程放疗[q]）

局部复发 → 不能切除 → 最佳支持治疗（KPS差；化疗[j]；或考虑再程放疗[q]）

第一章 高级别胶质细胞肿瘤

a 包括间变性少突-星形细胞瘤（AOA）、间变性星形细胞瘤（AA）、间变性少突胶质细胞瘤（AO）和其他少见间变性胶质细胞瘤。
b 若MRI考虑肿瘤为原发性中枢神经系统淋巴瘤，则首先活检。
c 制订治疗计划时，考虑多学科综合治疗，特别是一旦获得病理诊断后。
d 保护神经功能的前提下最大范围的切除肿瘤，立体定向活检或开颅活检。
e 如果术中冰冻病理切片支持高级别胶质细胞瘤。
f BCNU植入片治疗可能会影响某些辅助治疗临床试验的入组。
g 术后在72小时内进行MRI复查。
h 包括胶质肉瘤。
i 见脑肿瘤放疗方案。
j 见脑肿瘤化疗方案。
k BCNU植入片治疗、再程放疗或多重初始全身化疗，可能会影响某些辅助临床试验的入组。
l 联合化疗药物可能会增加毒性或引起影像学上改变。
m GBM超过6个月的替莫唑胺辅助化疗是否获益不清楚，间变性胶质细胞瘤替莫唑胺辅助化疗持续时间尚不清楚。
n 考虑行MR波谱分析，MR灌注成像，或脑PET检查排除放射性坏死。
o 放疗和同期替莫唑胺化疗结束后头3个月内，肿瘤的复发与假性进展在神经影像学上难以鉴别。如果是假性进展，放疗结束后的3个月内，肿瘤症状可稳定或改善。
p 间变性少突胶质细胞瘤对化疗特别敏感，替莫唑胺或亚硝基脲类为基础化疗方案是合适的。
q 特别是放疗后肿瘤无进展期长和/或既往放疗效果好者。

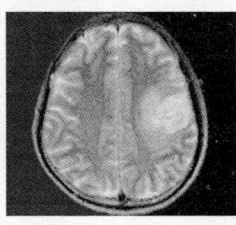

第二章
低级别侵润性胶质细胞瘤

Invasive low-grade gliomas

低级别浸润性胶质细胞瘤

弥漫性浸润性低级别胶质细胞瘤包括星形细胞瘤、少突胶质细胞瘤、少突-星形细胞瘤,属于WHO分类Ⅱ级肿瘤。低级别胶质细胞瘤是一种分化较好的肿瘤,但多数呈浸润性生长。低级别星形细胞瘤通常在病理形态极为相似的情况下,其生物学行为和预后相差很大。其中弥漫性星形细胞瘤(纤维型、原浆型和肥胖型细胞性星形细胞瘤)占70%,多呈浸润性生长,可转化为高级别星形细胞瘤。大脑胶质细胞瘤病的特点是广泛弥散性生长,侵犯多个脑叶。毛细胞型星形细胞瘤是最常见的非浸润性星形细胞瘤,常呈局限性生长,可通过单纯手术达到治愈,且一般不转化为高级别星形细胞瘤。其他比较少见的低级别胶质细胞瘤还包括多形性黄色星形细胞瘤、室管膜下巨细胞星形细胞瘤。少突胶质细胞瘤在影像学上表现为界限清楚、常伴有钙化、无对比增强等特征。在组织病理学上,其"蜂窝样"征象在石蜡切片中较为明显,而在冰冻切片中较难发现。超过半数的少突胶质细胞瘤存在染色体1p/19q杂合性缺失,此特征有助于鉴别诊断。WHOⅡ级的少突胶质细胞瘤、少突-星形细胞瘤和星形细胞瘤的5年生存率分别为70%、56%和37%。

癫痫发作(66%)与头痛是低级别胶质细胞瘤最常见的临床表现。从出现症状到诊断的中位时间为6~17个月。发病中位年龄为37岁。年龄是影响预后的最重要因素。不利预后因素包括:年龄≥40岁,星形细胞瘤病理类型,肿瘤直径≥6cm,肿瘤超过中线,手术前已出现神经功能缺失症状。具有≤2个不利预后因素的患者被认为是低危患者,具有≥3个不

第二章 低级别浸润性胶质细胞瘤

利预后因素的患者认为是高危患者。儿童的10年总生存率达83%，而大于40岁患者的中位生存时间仅为5年。其他可能的、有利的预后因素包括症状持续时间长、术后良好的神经功能状态及增殖指数（labeling index，LI）低等。在CT/MR中常表现为不强化或低强化病灶。然而影像诊断低级别胶质细胞瘤有25%的误诊率。

虽然低级别胶质细胞瘤通常被认为是良性肿瘤，但其中有许多肿瘤尽管采用手术和分次外照射放疗后仍有侵袭性生长。经过5～10年后可能转变为恶性胶质细胞瘤。对于伴有癫痫发作的低级别胶质细胞瘤患者的最佳治疗策略目前尚无定论。一般认为，应尽可能切除肿瘤，因其与患者的生存及复发时间相关。此外，全切除肿瘤有可能延迟或阻止其向恶性肿瘤转变。当然有些浸润性肿瘤及侵及功能区的肿瘤是无法达到完全切除的。

手术是低级别胶质细胞瘤诊断及治疗最重要的手段。手术目的是全切除肿瘤，获取足够的组织标本进行病理诊断及分级。当肿瘤位于较深部位或功能区时，可使用立体定向活检。由于肿瘤组织各区域内细胞的构成、细胞增殖水平及坏死情况可能不一致，因此活检也可能导致不准确的诊断。

术后放疗的时机目前暂无统一认识。部分学者提倡术后立即行分次外照射，但也有观点认为术后可先行观察，待肿瘤进展再予以放疗，因为有研究表明，术后早期放疗与肿瘤复发后放疗患者的总生存期在统计学上无显著差异。放疗剂量多为45～54Gy，分割剂量为1.8～2Gy/次。

目前，替莫唑胺也是低级别胶质细胞瘤治疗中可考虑选择的药物。对复发进展患者，仍可选择化疗，包括替莫唑胺、亚硝基脲类药物、PCV方案、铂类为基础的方案等。低级别少突胶质细胞瘤特别是伴有染色体1p/19q杂合性缺失者，更适合选择化疗。

成人幕上浸润性低级别星形细胞瘤/少突胶质细胞瘤（除外毛细胞型星形细胞瘤）

诊疗流程

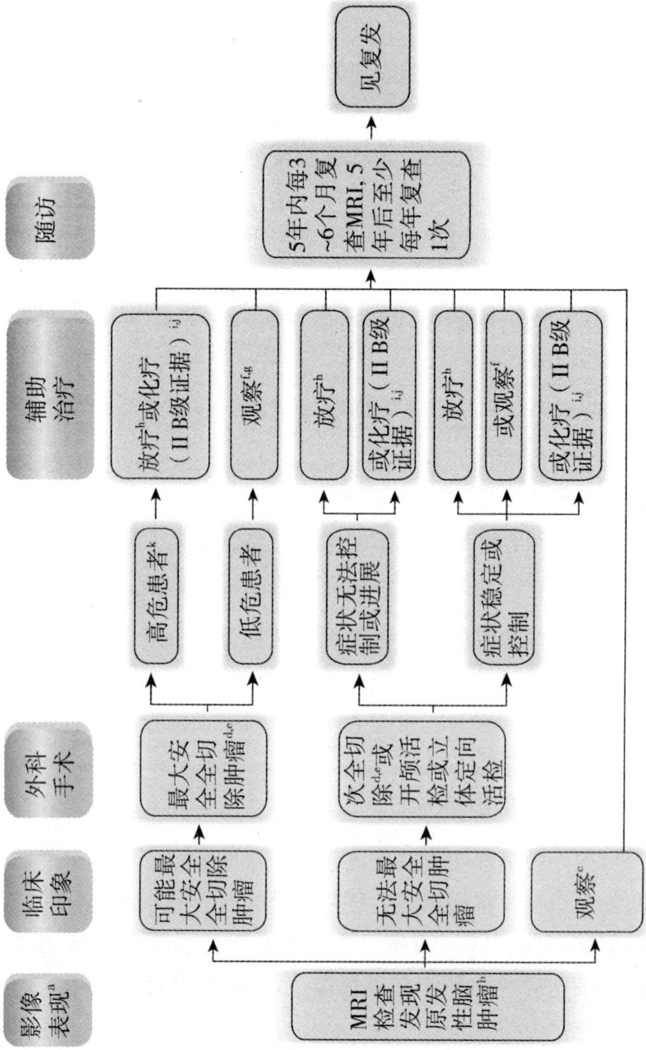

影像表现：MRI检查发现原发性脑肿瘤[a]

临床印象：
- 可能最大安全切除肿瘤
- 无法最大安全切肿瘤
- 观察[c]

外科手术：
- 最大安全切除肿瘤[c,d,e]
- 次全切除[d,e]或开颅活检或立体定向活检

术后评估：
- 高危患者[k] → 放疗[h]或化疗（ⅡB级证据）[i,j]
- 低危患者 → 观察[f,g]
- 症状无法控制或进展 → 放疗[h]或化疗（ⅡB级证据）[i,j]
- 症状稳定或控制 → 放疗[h]或观察或化疗（ⅡB级证据）[i,j]

随访：5年内每3~6个月复查MRI，5年后至少每年复查1次 → 见复发

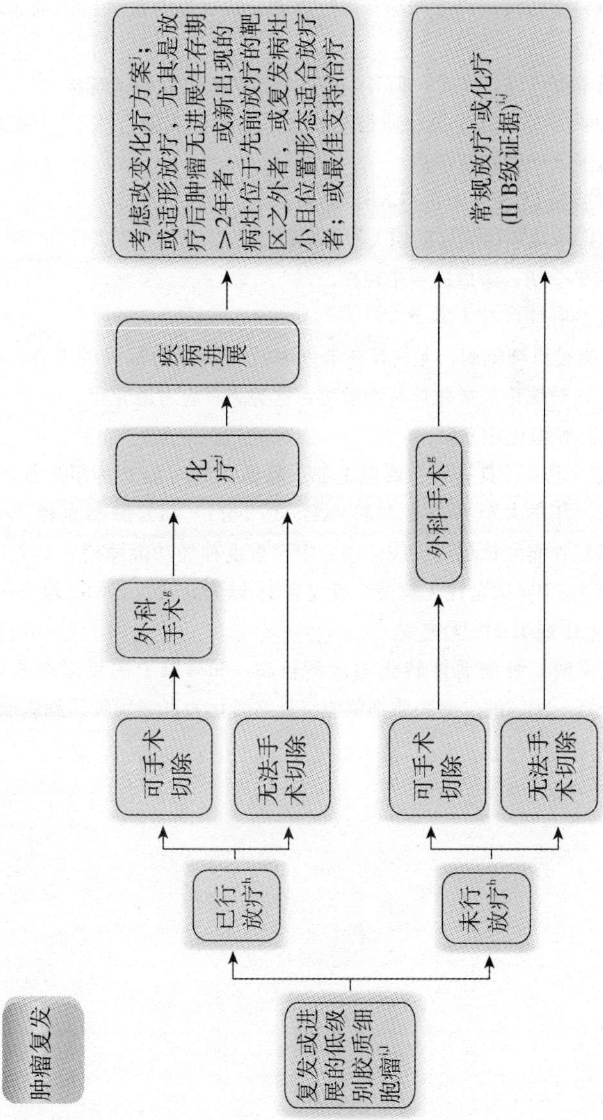

第二章 低级别浸润性胶质细胞瘤

肿瘤复发

复发或进展的低级别胶质瘤[i,j]
→ 已行放疗[h] → 可手术切除 → 外科手术[g] → 化疗 → 疾病进展 → 考虑改变化疗方案；或适形放疗，尤其是放疗后肿瘤无进展生存期>2年者，或新出现的病灶位于先前放疗的靶区之外者，或复发病灶小且位置适合放疗者；或最佳支持治疗
　　　　　　　　　无法手术切除 → 化疗 ↗

复发或进展的低级别胶质瘤[i,j]
→ 未行放疗[h] → 可手术切除 → 外科手术[g] → 常规放疗[h]或化疗 (ⅡB级证据)[i,j]
　　　　　　　　　无法手术切除 ↗

a 根据脑肿瘤影像检查判断。
b 制订治疗计划时考虑综合治疗原则,特别是一旦获得明确病理诊断后。
c 通常推荐外科手术,但对一些选择性病人可以系统观察。
d 如果肿瘤中有少突胶质细胞成分,考虑检测染色体 1p/19q 缺失状况,帮助判断预后。
e 术后在 72 小时内进行 MRI 复查。
f 术后单纯随访观察的病人应规律随访。
g 如果全切,考虑进一步观察。
h 见脑肿瘤放疗方案。
i 少突胶质细胞瘤,尤其存在染色体 1p/19q 联合缺失的患者,有报道其对烷化剂类化疗药物敏感,这类患者应考虑化疗。
j 见脑肿瘤化疗方案。
k 高危患者:具有 3 个或以上如下特征:(1)病理为星形细胞瘤;(2)年龄大于 40 岁;(3)KPS<70 分;(4)肿瘤直径>6cm;(5)肿瘤生长越过中线;(6)中至重度神经功能障碍;(7)染色体 1p/19q 杂合性无缺失,或仅有 1p 缺失,或仅有 19q 缺失;(8)IDH1 或 IDH2 无突变。
l 复发时,肿瘤恶性转化的比例较高,60% 以上的星形细胞瘤和 40%~50% 的少突胶质细胞瘤将最终转化为高级别胶质细胞瘤。

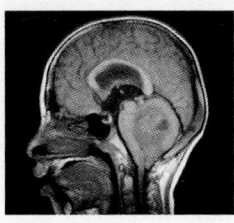

第三章

室管膜瘤和间变性室管膜瘤

室管膜瘤和间变性室管膜瘤

室管膜瘤可发生于成人和儿童。在成人，33%的室管膜瘤发生于幕下，66%发生于幕上，而儿童正好相反，以幕下为主。肿瘤可引起脑积水、颅内高压、脑干受压，引起颅神经麻痹、局灶性小脑神经功能缺失等症状，如果侵犯颈髓上部，常可导致颈部僵硬和斜颈。

室管膜瘤的预后与手术切除程度密切相关，肿瘤全切的患者预后较好。如果手术切除不完全，即使是低级别的室管膜瘤，预后也不良。放疗可以明显提高肿瘤控制率和延长生存时间。术后辅助放疗患者的 5 年生存率为 33%～80%。幕上室管膜瘤多为高级别，且不易手术全切，术后常有病灶残留，故预后较幕下室管膜瘤患者差。

儿童室管膜瘤脑脊液播散相对较少。有临床研究显示，接受局部放疗患者的预后与全中枢放疗相当，因此，是否仅做后颅窝放疗是目前争议的热点。对于间变性室管膜瘤，尽管不十分确定，也有资料显示局部放疗一样可行。室管膜瘤常规放疗剂量为总量 54～60Gy，1.8～2.0Gy/次。

间变性室管膜瘤伴脑脊膜播散者推荐全中枢放疗，加局部病灶追加剂量放疗。值得注意的是，研究证实：1. 室管膜瘤治疗失败的主要原因为局部复发；2. 局部未复发的患者较少出现脊髓播散；3. 无论采取局部放疗或全中枢放疗，高级别肿瘤治疗失败的原因相似；4. 预防性治疗也许不能防止脊髓播撒转移。因此，常规采用"预防性"全中枢或全脑放疗不一定能提高生存率。Ⅱ级和Ⅲ级的室管膜瘤患者采用手术/放疗综合治疗的 5 年生存率约为 70%。

第三章 室管膜瘤和间变性室管膜瘤

化疗在室管膜瘤治疗中的作用还不确定。目前的研究显示室管膜瘤对化疗并不十分敏感，对于儿童或成人新诊断的室管膜瘤，无临床研究证实化疗联合放疗与单纯放疗比较对生存率有改善。但对于复发进展型患者，化疗可作为挽救治疗，化疗药物包括 VP-16、替莫唑胺、亚硝脲类、铂类等。

成人室管膜瘤的治疗策略需根据组织病理学类型、手术切除程度、肿瘤播散程度等综合考虑。为避免术后人为干扰和假阳性结果，应于术后 2～3 周复查脊髓 MRI，应在术后 2 周做腰椎穿刺脑脊液检查。肿瘤全切除、分化良好、脊髓 MRI 检查阴性的患者，推荐局部放疗或观察（仅幕上肿瘤）。幕下肿瘤也可考虑放疗或观察，但如果脊髓 MRI 增强扫描或脑脊液检查阳性，建议行全中枢放疗。

间变性室管膜瘤患者在活检或次全切除后应行脑脊髓 MRI 增强扫描和脑脊液检查。如果 MRI 阴性，推荐局部放疗：临床靶区为肿瘤体积加上边缘 1～2cm，总剂量 54.0～59.4Gy，1.8～2.0Gy/次。如果 MRI 或脑脊液检查阳性，推荐全中枢放疗：全脑全脊髓剂量 36Gy，1.8Gy/次，脊髓局部病灶剂量 45Gy，脑原发病灶剂量 54.0～59.4Gy，1.8～2.0Gy/次。室管膜瘤患者的随访间隔根据肿瘤的部位和范围而定：局限于术后 2～3 周复查脑和脊髓 MRI 增强扫描（如果术前为阳性），术后第 1 年每 3～4 个月复查 1 次，第 2 年每 4～6 个月复查 1 次，以后每半年至 1 年复查 1 次，具体根据医生针对肿瘤的病理类型和其他有关因素的判断而定。影像学检查提示复发者，如果适合手术，尽量以手术切除之，手术后再加局部放疗（如果以前未放疗过）；如果不适合手术，以前未放疗过，则应考虑行放疗（包括合适部位的立体定向放疗）；也可考虑化疗（但无随机对照临床研究证实）或最佳支持疗法，取决于肿瘤的病理类型、肿瘤范围、患者年龄和 KPS 状态。放疗（包括合适部位的立体定向放疗）对于手术后复发患者也可予以考虑。

成人颅内室管膜瘤

诊 疗 流 程

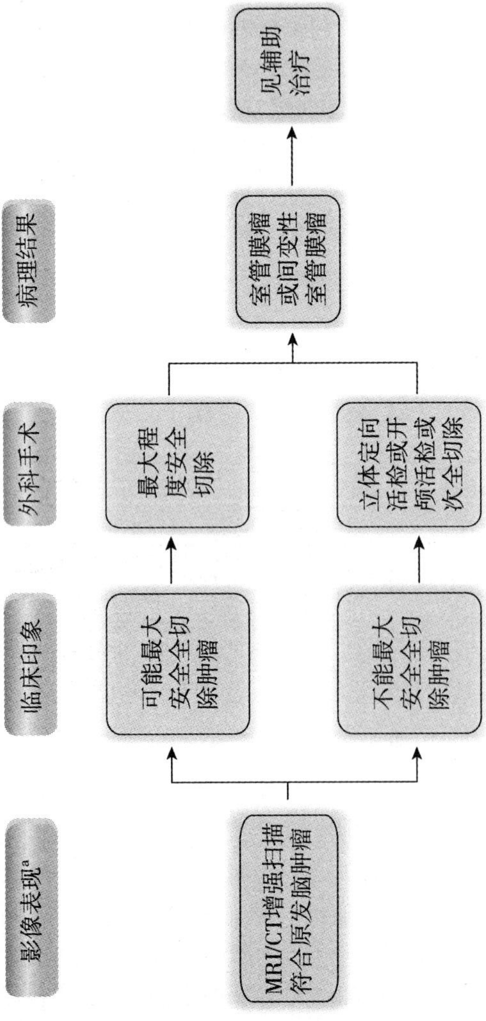

影像表现[a]	临床印象	外科手术	病理结果	
MRI/CT增强扫描符合原发脑肿瘤	可能最大安全切除肿瘤	最大程度安全切除	室管膜瘤或间变性室管膜瘤	见辅助治疗
	不能最大安全切除肿瘤	立体定向活检或开颅活检或次全切除		

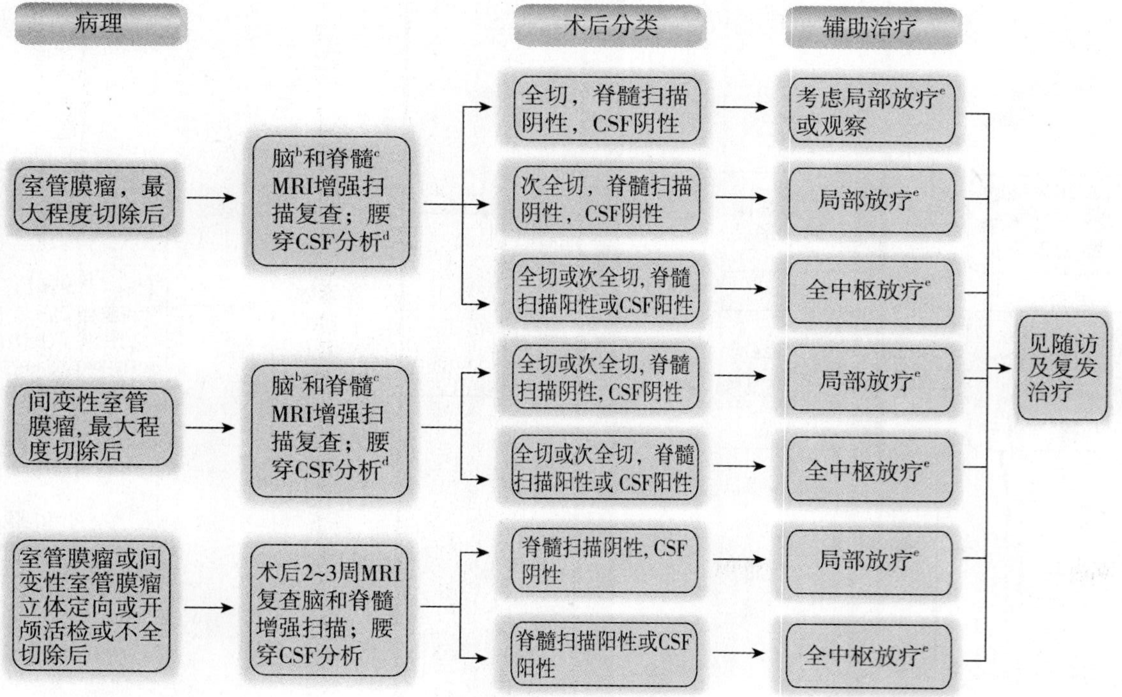

第三章 室管膜瘤和间变性室管膜瘤

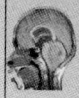

病理		术后分类	辅助治疗
室管膜瘤,最大程度切除后	脑[b]和脊髓MRI增强扫描复查;腰穿CSF分析[d]	全切,脊髓扫描阴性,CSF阴性	考虑局部放疗[e]或观察
		次全切,脊髓扫描阴性,CSF阴性	局部放疗[e]
		全切或次全切,脊髓扫描阳性或CSF阳性	全中枢放疗[e]
间变性室管膜瘤,最大程度切除后	脑[b]和脊髓MRI增强扫描复查;腰穿CSF分析[d]	全切或次全切,脊髓扫描阴性,CSF阴性	局部放疗[e]
		全切或次全切,脊髓扫描阳性或CSF阳性	全中枢放疗[e]
室管膜瘤或间变性室管膜瘤立体定向或开颅活检或不全切除后	术后2~3周MRI复查脑和脊髓增强扫描;腰穿CSF分析	脊髓扫描阴性,CSF阴性	局部放疗[e]
		脊髓扫描阴性或CSF阳性	全中枢放疗[e]

→ 见随访复发治疗

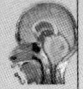

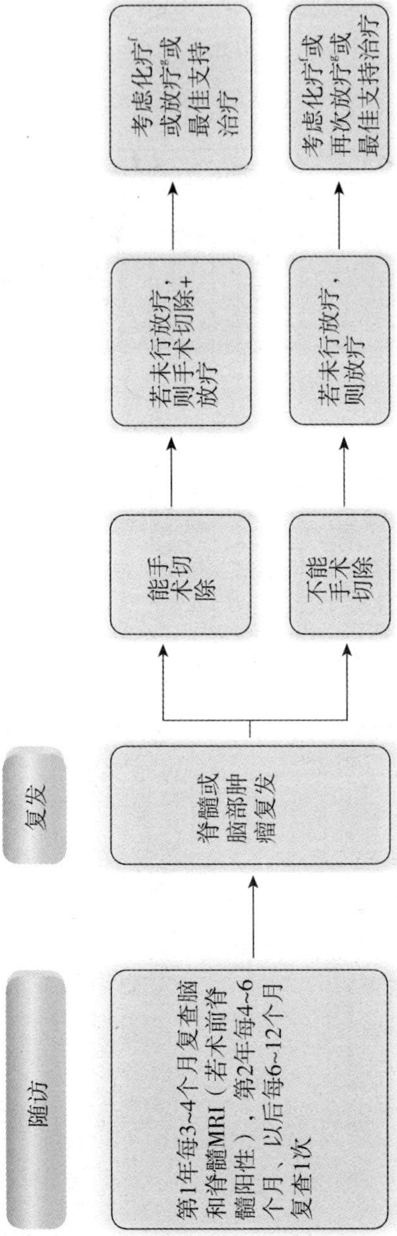

中枢神经系统常见肿瘤诊疗纲要

随访：第1年每3~4个月复查脑和脊髓MRI（若术前脊髓阳性），第2年每4~6个月，以后每6~12个月复查1次

复发：脊髓或脑部肿瘤复发

- 能手术切除 → 若未行放疗，则手术切除+放疗 → 考虑化疗或放疗或最佳支持治疗
- 不能手术切除 → 若未行放疗，则放疗 → 考虑化疗或再次放疗或最佳支持治疗

a 根据脑肿瘤影像检查判断。
b 在 24~72h 内复查。
c 术后 2~3 周行脊髓 MRI 复查以避免术后人为干扰。
d 术后至少 2 周后才进行腰椎穿刺检查以避免可能的假阳性结果。
e 见脑肿瘤放疗方案。
f 见脑肿瘤化疗方案。
g 如果肿瘤形态、大小合适,可考虑立体定向放射治疗(SRS)。

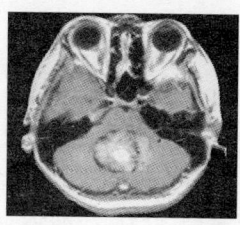

第四章

髓母细胞瘤/中枢神经系统原始神经外胚层肿瘤

Medulloblastoma / central nervous system primitive neuroectodermal tumor

髓母细胞瘤/中枢神经系统原始神经外胚层肿瘤

髓母细胞瘤是一种胚胎性肿瘤，多起源于小脑的下蚓部，发生于幕上者又称为原始神经外胚层肿瘤（primitive neuroectodermal tumours，PNETs）。85%的病例在15岁以前发病，约占所有儿童脑和脊髓肿瘤的20%。临床上患者常表现为颅内高压和小脑症状，肿瘤压迫第Ⅳ脑室所致的颅内高压症状比小脑的症状更常见。手术切除肿瘤是基本治疗方法，力求全切肿瘤，并要解除脑脊液循环障碍。颅内高压紧急情况下往往需要先行脑室外引流术。

髓母细胞瘤可沿小脑脚侵犯第四脑室，沿脑脊液播散到脊髓和天幕上颅腔。初诊时脑脊液肿瘤种植的发生率约为10%~40%。治疗前需要做全身检查和脑与脊髓MRI扫描，情况允许下应做腰椎穿刺并行脑脊液细胞学检查，明确肿瘤范围。术前颅内高压不能行腰椎穿刺脑脊液检查者，术后14天左右须行此检查。

术前进行分期诊断的目的是了解肿瘤有无转移/播散，为制订治疗策略提供证据。目前较常用的是Chang氏术前分期：M_0肿瘤局限，无转移证据；M_1脑脊液检查镜下找到瘤细胞；M_2颅内结节状种植；M_3脊髓结节状种植；M_4颅外转移。

髓母细胞瘤的临床治疗常根据术前分期和手术后肿瘤残留情况综合考虑。术后需要进行头颅MRI检查，将患者分为中危和高危两组进行不同的治疗。中危：肿瘤全切除或者近全切除，残留病灶小于1.5cm，无扩散转移。高危：年龄<3岁，或病理类型为大细胞/间变型，或肿瘤次全切除，残留病灶大于1.5cm，或非后颅窝定位，即幕上原始神经外胚叶肿瘤。目前探索的治疗方案是对中危患者降低治疗的强度，高危患者则

第四章 髓母细胞瘤/中枢神经系统原始神经外胚层肿瘤

增加治疗强度。

中危髓母细胞瘤患者手术后全中枢放疗 36Gy,后颅窝追加 18~20 Gy,5 年无进展生存约为 50%~65%。然而,生存患者存在放疗所致的智力下降、生长迟缓、内分泌功能障碍与听力下降,继发肿瘤发生率大约 12%,因此,探讨在中危髓母细胞瘤患者治疗过程中减低放疗剂量,减少放疗所致后遗症的发生是目前研究的重点。手术后全中枢降低剂量放疗后联合化疗,是目前 3 岁以上中危髓母细胞瘤患者标准治疗的方案。具体是术后 28 天内行放疗,全中枢 23.4Gy,后颅窝追加 31.8Gy,放疗结束后 6 周,进行辅助化疗,药物为长春新碱、顺铂和洛莫司汀,每 6 周 1 疗程,共 8 个疗程。此方案的 5 年无进展生存率约为 79%。也有推荐放疗期间每周静脉注射长春新碱 $1.5mg/m^2$(最大剂量 2mg)。

高危髓母细胞瘤如按中危髓母细胞瘤的治疗策略,其 5 年生存率低于 55%,但是松果体区 PNET 的预后比其他幕上 PNET 要好,5 年生存率可达 70%。高危髓母细胞瘤患者在手术/放疗基础上需增加化疗剂量强度,有条件者推荐行自体造血干细胞支持下的超大剂量化疗,5 年生存率获得改善可达 70%。目前推荐大于 3 岁高危髓母细胞瘤患者的治疗方法为:手术联合标准剂量放疗,即全中枢放疗剂量 36~39Gy,瘤床总剂量为 55.8Gy;放疗结束后 6 周,进行辅助化疗,有条件者可联合自体造血干细胞支持下的超大剂量化疗。

对小于 3 岁的髓母细胞瘤患者无论术后有无肿瘤残留,均定义为高危。一般不主张术后马上放疗,因为放疗对小于 3 岁患儿的生长发育影响较大。手术联合化疗仍能使部分患者获得较好的疗效。如果手术能完全切除或化疗获得完全缓解的患儿,可考虑推迟放疗或调整放疗剂量或不进行放疗,若肿瘤复发则再行放疗。有效的化疗药物包括环磷酰胺、长春新碱、依托泊苷、顺铂和洛莫司汀等。

髓母细胞瘤/幕上原始神经外胚层肿瘤[a]

诊疗流程

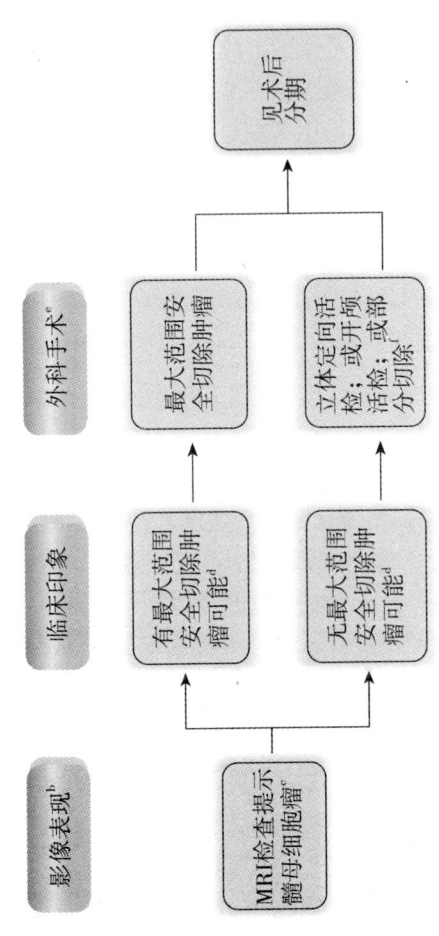

影像表现[b]: MRI检查提示髓母细胞瘤[c]

临床印象: 有最大范围安全切除肿瘤可能[d] / 无最大范围安全切除肿瘤可能[d]

外科手术[e]: 最大范围安全切除肿瘤 / 立体定向活检；或开颅活检；或部分切除

→ 见术后分期

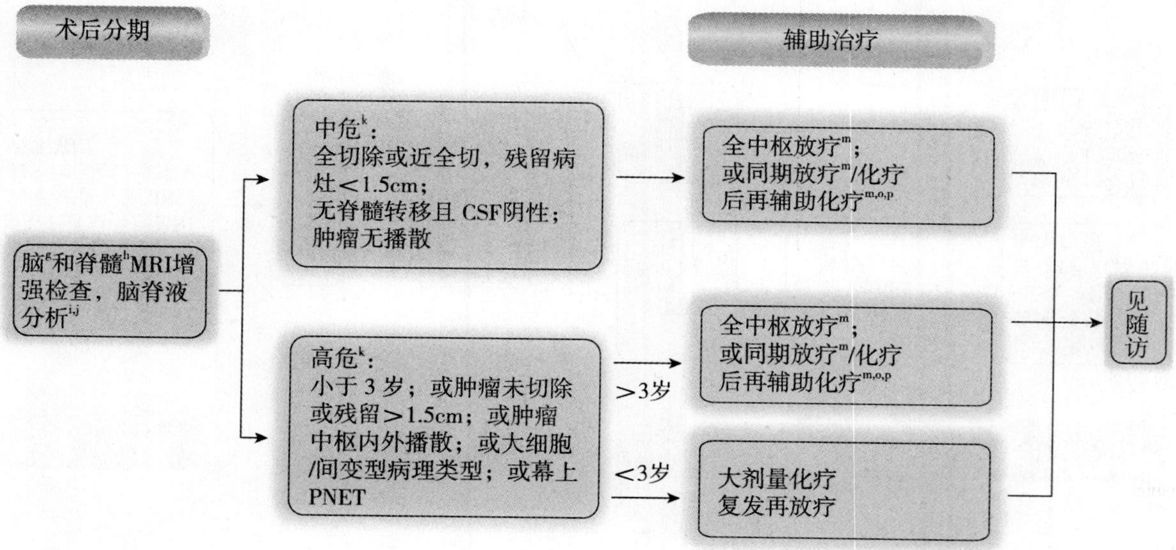

第四章 髓母细胞瘤/中枢神经系统原始神经外胚层肿瘤

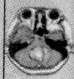

术后分期

脑和脊髓 MRI 增强检查，脑脊液分析[j]

↓

中危[k]：
全切除或近全切，残留病灶 <1.5cm；无脊髓转移且 CSF 阴性；肿瘤无播散

高危[k]：
小于 3 岁；或肿瘤未切除或残留 >1.5cm；或肿瘤中枢内外播散；或大细胞/间变型病理类型；或幕上 PNET

辅助治疗

全中枢放疗[m]；或同期放疗/化疗[m,o,p] 后再辅助化疗 → 见随访

>3岁 → 全中枢放疗[m]；或同期放疗/化疗[m,o,p] 后再辅助化疗 → 见随访

<3岁 → 大剂量化疗复发后再放疗 → 见随访

27

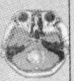中枢神经系统常见肿瘤诊疗纲要

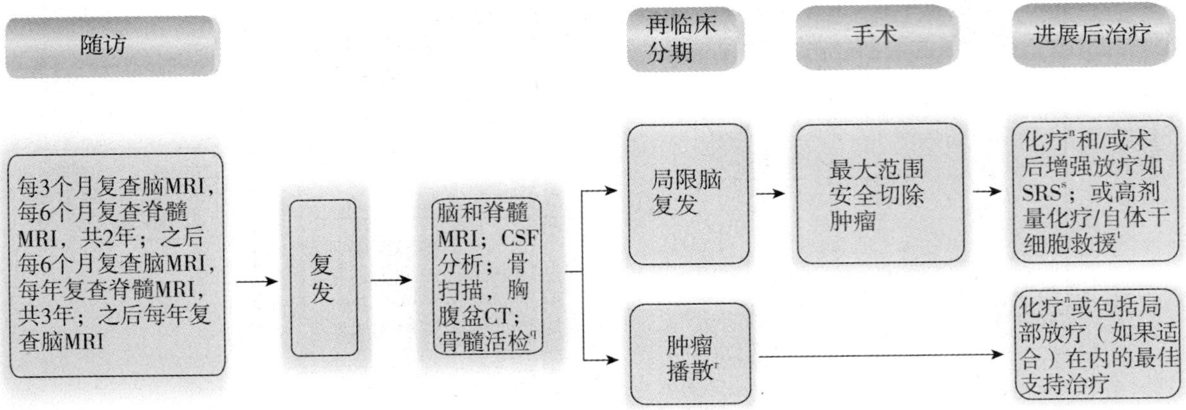

| 随访 | | 再临床分期 | 手术 | 进展后治疗 |

随访：每3个月复查脑MRI，每6个月复查脊髓MRI，共2年；之后每6个月复查脑MRI，每年复查脊髓MRI，共3年；之后每年复查脑MRI

↓

复发

↓

脑和脊髓MRI；CSF分析；骨扫描，胸腹盆CT；骨髓活检⁽¹⁾

↓ ↓

局限脑复发 → 最大范围安全切除肿瘤 → 化疗和/或术后增强放疗如SRS；或高剂量化疗自体干细胞救援

肿瘤播散 → 化疗⁽²⁾或包括局部放疗（如果适合）在内的最佳支持治疗

28

第四章 髓母细胞瘤/中枢神经系统原始神经外胚层肿瘤

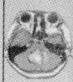

a 除外松果体母细胞瘤和嗅神经母细胞瘤。
b 根据髓母细胞瘤影像学检查特征判断。
c 术前和一旦获得明确病理诊断后,在制订治疗计划时考虑多学科综合治疗原则。
d 如果临床需要,可放置脑室-腹腔分流管。
e 保护神经功能的前提下最大范围的切除肿瘤,立体定向活检或开颅活检。
f 强烈推荐患者至大型神经肿瘤中心做进一步评估,争取更完全的手术切除。
g 24~72 小时内。
h 脊髓 MRI 检查推迟到术后至少 2~3 周,以避免术后干扰。
i 脊髓 MRI 检查后行腰穿检查,术后至少 2 周行腰穿脑脊液检查,以避免假阳性。
j 骨扫描,胸、腹、盆 CT,骨髓活检等检查仅用于有临床征象时。
k 见髓母细胞瘤 Chang 氏分期系统。
l 若仅行活检,可考虑先行放疗和化疗后再手术切除。
m 见脑肿瘤放疗方案。
n 见脑肿瘤化疗方案。
o 成人髓母细胞瘤放疗期间可不用长春新碱,可调整化疗剂量,因为成人对髓母细胞瘤化疗方案耐受性差,放疗期间同步用长春新碱的资料仅来自儿童患者的临床试验中。儿童患者应定期检查监测放疗/化疗可能所致的神经毒性。
p 推荐铂类为基础的化疗。
q 有临床症状时检查。如果病人初治时仅行单纯放疗,复发时骨扫描应作为再分期的手段之一,即使患者无临床症状。
r 考虑姑息减症手术。
s 伽玛刀补充放疗剂量治疗。
t 大剂量化疗/自体干细胞救援仅用于患者在手术后或传统剂量再诱导化疗后肿瘤完全缓解时。

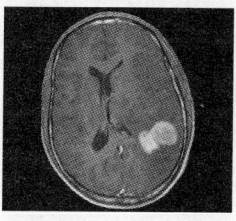

第五章
原发性中枢神经系统淋巴瘤

原发性中枢神经系统淋巴瘤

原发性中枢神经系统淋巴瘤（primary central nervous system lymphoma，PCNSL）是一种侵袭性非霍奇金淋巴瘤，可发生于脑、脊髓、眼及软脑膜。在所有脑肿瘤中PCNSL占约0.5%~2%。近20年，无论是免疫抑制性还是非免疫抑制性中枢神经系统淋巴瘤的发病率都有明显的升高。在非免疫抑制性患者中，平均诊断年龄是55岁；免疫抑制性患者则较为年轻，在艾滋病患者中平均诊断年龄为31岁。

PCNSL好发于幕上、脑室旁，小脑和脑干也可见到，软脑膜和脊髓较少发生。临床表现：超过50%患者表现为局部神经系统功能障碍（如轻偏瘫、言语困难）；33%患者出现智力下降（记忆力下降或紊乱）及颅内高压症状（头痛、呕吐）；癫痫发作较少见，约为10%；眼部受侵可出现视物模糊或视物成漂浮状；脊髓受侵患者常有颈部或肩背部疼痛。

立体定向活检是明确病理诊断的最佳选择。此病以多病灶为特点，广泛的切除不但可能降低生存率，且有加大术后神经功能障碍的风险。

放疗在PCNSL治疗中的地位不断提升。目前推荐在大剂量MTX方案化疗基础上行全脑放疗，剂量为全脑24~36Gy，1.8~2Gy/次，不需要缩野加量。为了避免放疗毒性反应，超过60岁的患者如果化疗后肿瘤消退不推荐行放疗，复发后再行局部放疗，剂量为46~50Gy。单纯放疗可行全脑照射36~40Gy，然后缩野肿瘤病灶总剂量为46~56Gy。眼部淋巴瘤患者可考虑选择放疗。对脊髓MRI阳性且CSF也阳性的患者，脊髓播散诊断明确，均应行全中枢轴放疗。

化疗方面，通常以大剂量甲氨蝶呤（HD-MTX）为基础的化疗方案优于其他方案，该方案使PCNSL患者无进展生存率及总生存率均明显得到改善。行单纯放疗者的中位生存期仅为12个月，联合化疗后可提高到30~51个月。

第五章 原发性中枢神经系统淋巴瘤

原发性中枢神经系统淋巴瘤（PCNSL）（非免疫抑制性）诊疗流程

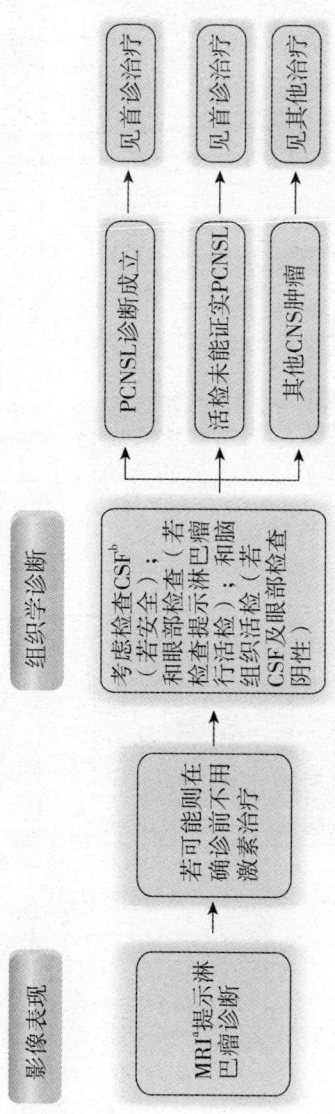

影像表现：MRI[a]提示淋巴瘤诊断 → 若可能则在确诊前不用激素治疗 → **组织学诊断**：考虑检查CSF[b]（若安全）；和眼部检查（若检查提示淋巴瘤行活检）；和脑组织活检（若CSF及眼部检查阴性）

- → PCNSL诊断成立 → 见首诊治疗
- → 活检未能证实PCNSL → 见首诊治疗
- → 其他CNS肿瘤 → 见其他治疗

中枢神经系统常见肿瘤诊疗纲要

疾病分期/诊断检查

裂隙灯检眼；
若无危险，行腰穿检查；
若有症状或CSF阳性行脊髓MRI；
HIV/胸片/CBC/血小板/肝功能检查；
胸腹盆腔CT（ⅡB）；
骨髓活检c（ⅡB）；
老年男性考虑睾丸超声检查；
考虑PET检查d,e

↓

- KPS≥40f,g且肌酐清除率≥50ml/min
- KPS<40f,g且肌酐清除率<50ml/min

首诊治疗

KPS≥40且肌酐清除率≥50ml/min：
HD-MTX为基础的化疗方案h,i ± 化疗结束后的全脑放疗j,k；
若CSF阳性或脊髓MRI阳性，考虑鞘内化疗；
若眼科检查阳性，则行眼内化疗（ⅡB）或眼球放疗

KPS<40且肌酐清除率<50ml/min：
全脑放疗；若眼科检查阳性，则行眼球放疗或考虑眼内化疗，若腰穿检查阳性可考虑鞘内化疗或脊髓MRI阳性可考虑鞘内化疗或脊髓局部放疗或者化疗l,m

---

诊断为PCNSL

活检未能证实PCNSL
- 已行激素治疗 → 停用激素治疗而当疾病进展时再次活检
- 未行激素治疗 → 行其他CNS疾病诊断检查或者再次活检

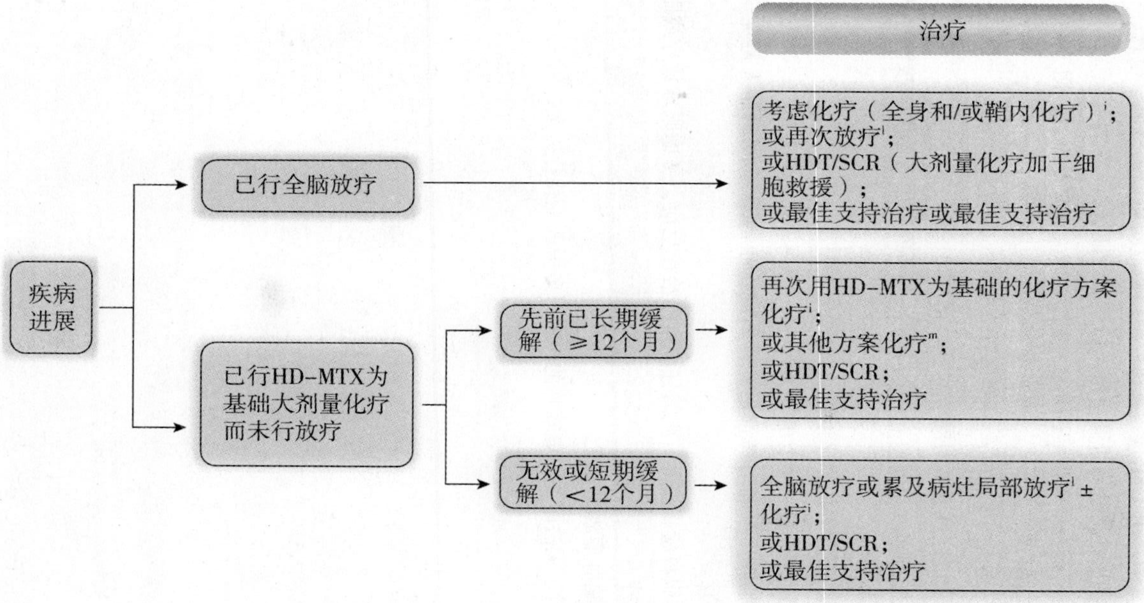

第五章 原发性中枢神经系统淋巴瘤

治疗

```
疾病进展
 ├── 已行全脑放疗 → 考虑化疗（全身和/或鞘内化疗）[1]；
 │                  或再次放疗；
 │                  或HDT/SCR（大剂量化疗加干细胞救援）；
 │                  或最佳支持治疗或最佳支持治疗
 │
 └── 已行HD-MTX为基础大剂量化疗而未行放疗
        ├── 先前已长期缓解（≥12个月） → 再次用HD-MTX为基础的化疗方案化疗[II]；
        │                                 或其他方案化疗[III]；
        │                                 或HDT/SCR；
        │                                 或最佳支持治疗
        │
        └── 无效或短期缓解（<12个月） → 全脑放疗或累及病灶局部放疗[I]±化疗[I]；
                                         或HDT/SCR；
                                         或最佳支持治疗
```

a 中枢 MRI 检查考虑为 CNS 淋巴瘤首先活检。
b 组织样本和 CSF 应包括流式细胞学检测和 CSF 细胞学检查。
c 一些医疗机构行骨髓活检，但还缺乏证据。
d PET 检查可取代 CT 检查、骨髓、睾丸超声检查，但用于 PCNSL 的资料缺乏。
e 适合所有 PCNSL 的分期指导。
f 激素治疗可以大大提高 KPS 评分。
g 年龄和评分指导尚未确立，医生有义务向患者阐明积极治疗的风险和获益。
h 强烈推荐参加临床试验。
i 见脑肿瘤常用化疗方案。
j 全脑放疗可能增加毒性，特别对于年龄＞60 岁的病人避免全脑放疗。
k 若眼科检查阳性，则需仔细监测治疗反应。考虑眼球放疗或眼内化疗。
l 见脑肿瘤放疗方案。
m 对于无法耐受甲氨蝶呤的患者可考虑改变化疗方案。

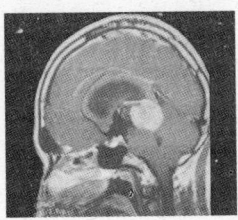

第六章

原发性中枢神经系统生殖细胞肿瘤

Primary central nervous system germ cell tumors

原发性中枢神经系统生殖细胞肿瘤

原发性中枢神经系统生殖细胞肿瘤（germ cell tumors，GCTs）约占所有颅内肿瘤的2%～3%。亚洲国家发生率比西方国家高。好发于年轻人群，70%发生在10～24岁。病理主要分为两大类型：①生殖细胞瘤（germinoma），相当于颅外睾丸精原细胞瘤或卵巢的无性细胞瘤，无甲胎蛋白（AFP）或绒毛膜促性腺激素（β-hCG）升高；②非生殖细胞瘤性生殖细胞肿瘤（nongerminoma germ cell tumor，NGGCT），相当于颅外的非精原细胞瘤，包括畸胎瘤、胚胎性癌、内胚窦瘤（卵黄囊瘤）、绒毛膜上皮癌和混合型肿瘤，常伴有AFP或β-hCG升高。

诊断CNS GCTs，检测血清和脑脊液AFP、β-hCG和胎盘碱性磷酸酶（PLAP）水平具有重要临床意义。绒毛膜上皮细胞瘤和胚胎性癌肿瘤细胞分泌β-hCG；AFP则由胚胎性癌肿瘤细胞和内胚窦瘤细胞分泌；生殖细胞瘤细胞分泌PLAP。这些肿瘤标志物已成为生殖细胞肿瘤患者重要的治疗前评价指标，但不能决定准确的组织亚型。未成熟畸胎瘤或胚胎癌有时也分泌β-hCG和AFP。血清和脑脊液PLAP的升高提示肿瘤含有生殖细胞瘤成分。肿瘤标志物还可作为疗效观察和随访的指标。

CNS GCTs好发蝶鞍区和松果体部位，位于脑的中央，手术切除难度较大。临床上常根据血清和脑脊液肿瘤标志物升高或细胞学阳性、典型影像学和临床表现做出CNS GCTs的临床诊断。但是，如果脑脊液和血清肿瘤标志物正常，细胞学检查结果阴性，则应尽可能获得组织学诊断。由于CNS GCTs的异质性，准确的诊断对治疗选择具有重要意义，外科手术在获得组织学诊断方面起着非常重要的作用。内镜活检或立体定位穿刺活检是获得组织学诊断的方法之一。

生殖细胞瘤对放疗很敏感,单纯放疗的治愈率大于90%,对儿童患者可通过联合化疗减少放疗的剂量和范围。NGGCT对放疗敏感性较差,单纯放疗治愈率仅30%~40%,需要化疗、放疗或手术等综合治疗改善生存率。放疗包括局部放疗和全中枢放疗。头颅放射治疗对青少年影响较大,长期副作用包括智力下降、生长迟缓、内分泌功能失调和听力下降,继发肿瘤发生率大约12%。全中枢放疗(全脑脊髓)还可引起生长阻滞、骨髓抑制和生殖器官损伤。原发颅内的生殖细胞瘤与颅外生殖细胞瘤相似,对化疗较敏感。然而,采用单纯化疗治疗颅内的生殖细胞瘤复发率较高,5年复发率达48%。标准的治疗方法为局部原发肿瘤放疗45~50Gy联合全中枢放疗,5年生存率可达90%~100%。为了减少全中枢放疗所致的长期副作用,国外不少研究者进行减少放疗剂量和范围或联合化疗的探索:(1)减少放疗剂量或范围:局限型颅内生殖细胞瘤行低剂量全中枢放疗21Gy,局部追加脑室9Gy和原发肿瘤部位19.5Gy,7年无病存活94%。(2)化疗联合单纯局部瘤床放疗:对局限型生殖细胞瘤患者先化疗2个疗程(VP-16,卡铂,异环磷酰胺),随后仅行局部瘤床放疗40Gy,不做全中枢放疗,4年总生存率达100%,无病存活率为93.3%。(3)国际儿童肿瘤协会中枢神经系统生殖细胞瘤96方案:局限型生殖细胞瘤采用单纯放疗(全中枢24Gy+瘤床追加16Gy)或化疗联合局部放疗(化疗2疗程,随后局部放疗40Gy)。结果:单纯放疗5年无病存活率为91%,总生存率94%。化疗联合局部放疗5年无病存活率为85%,总生存率92%,脑室部位复发危险增加,新的方案则增加脑室部位放疗。对播散型生殖细胞瘤推荐行全中枢+局部放疗(瘤床和转移灶)。回顾性分析显示,化疗+局部放疗虽减少了放疗的范围,但颅内和脊髓转移的危险性明显高于全中枢放疗的患者。

NGGCT 与纯生殖细胞瘤相比预后较差，单纯放疗 5 年生存率为 10%～38%，需要手术、化疗和放疗等综合治疗来改善生存率。有研究显示：先行 3～4 个疗程化疗，然后接受全中枢及瘤床放疗，放疗后再化疗 4 个疗程，4 年无事件生存率达 67%～75%。国际儿童肿瘤协会中枢神经系统生殖细胞瘤 96 方案：先行 4 个疗程铂类为主化疗，随后施行肿瘤切除和放疗。放疗范围根据分期决定：局限型 NGGCT 化疗后局部放疗 54Gy，播散型患者行全中枢放疗 30Gy，瘤床追加 24Gy，约有 2/3 的患者获得长期生存。NGGCT 对化疗和放疗的敏感性均低于纯生殖细胞瘤，特别是恶性畸胎瘤，对于这一类型的肿瘤，尽可能首先手术切除，未能接受手术而行放、化疗后的残留病灶最好能手术切除，有助于改善生存率。

立体定向伽玛射线可精确定位杀灭肿瘤减少对周围正常组织的损伤，从而减少对下丘脑-垂体轴的影响，对青少年患者意义较大。然而，脑的恶性生殖细胞肿瘤具有侵袭性和转移性的行为，常沿脑室、脑脊髓通道转移至大脑、脑室和脊髓。单纯伽玛刀治疗脑恶性生殖细胞瘤，其复发、转移率高。伽玛刀治疗后复发和转移的患者，特别是多次伽玛刀治疗的患者，再次治疗难度较大，难以接受进一步放射治疗。如果这些患者首次治疗采用标准的治疗方案，则其生存率将会比单纯伽玛刀治疗要高。因此，伽玛刀治疗脑生殖细胞肿瘤应该联合其他治疗方法，作为综合治疗的一部分。

第六章 原发性中枢神经系统生殖细胞肿瘤

原发性中枢神经系统生殖细胞肿瘤诊疗流程

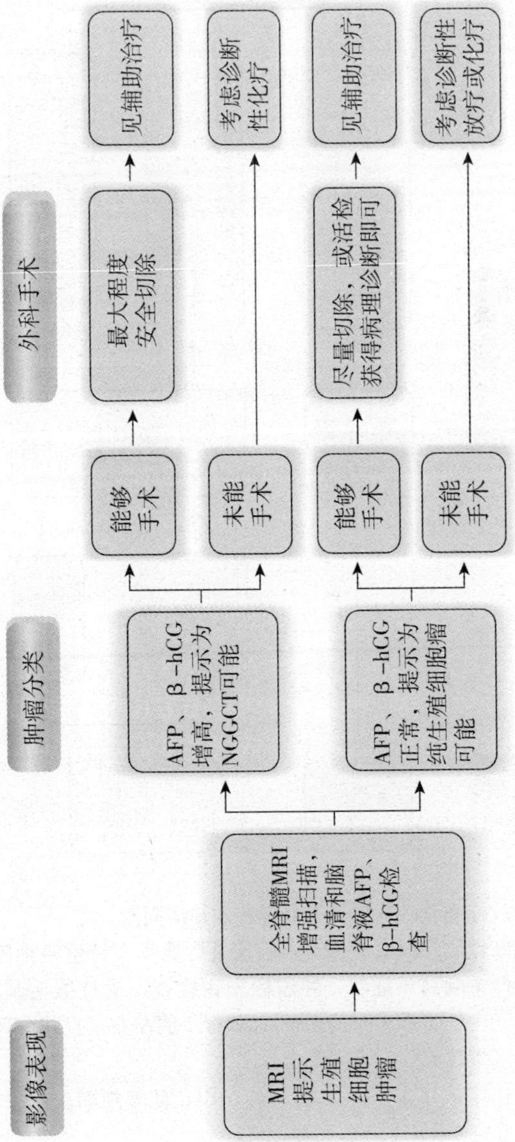

影像表现：MRI提示生殖细胞肿瘤 → 全脊髓MRI增强扫描，血清、脊液AFP、β-hCG检查

肿瘤分类：
- AFP、β-hCG增高，提示为NGGCT可能
- AFP、β-hCG正常，纯生殖细胞瘤可能

外科手术：
- 能够手术 → 最大程度安全切除 → 见辅助治疗
- 未能手术 → 考虑诊断性化疗
- 能够手术 → 尽量切除，获得病理诊断即可 → 见辅助治疗
- 未能手术 → 考虑诊断性放疗或化疗

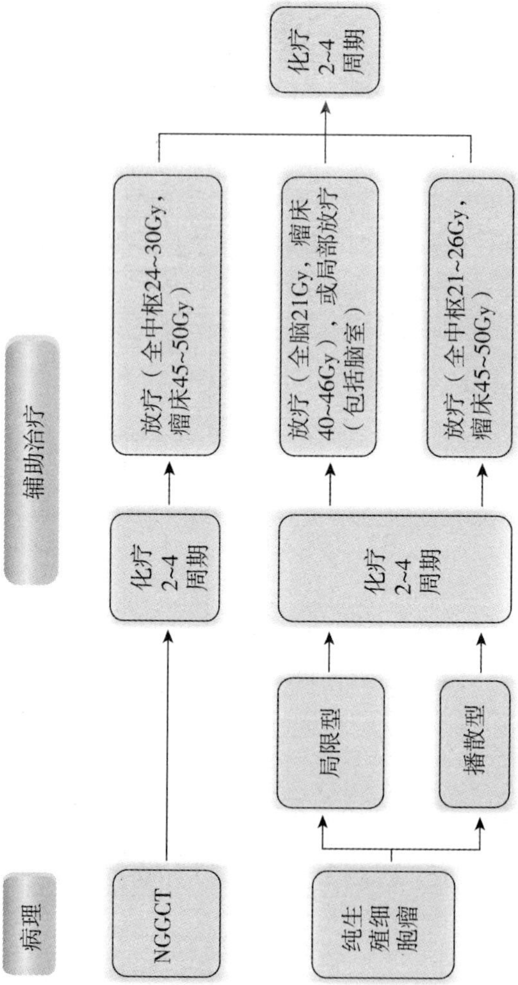

```
病理              辅助治疗

NGGCT → 化疗2~4周期 → 放疗（全中枢24~30Gy，瘤床45~50Gy）┐
                                                              │
                         局限型 → 化疗2~4周期 → 放疗（全脑21Gy，瘤床40~46Gy，或局部放疗（包括脑室））├→ 化疗2~4周期
纯生殖细胞瘤 ↗                                                 │
            ↘ 播散型 → 化疗2~4周期 → 放疗（全中枢21~26Gy，瘤床45~50Gy）┘
```

注：
1. 诊断性放疗和化疗需患者充分理解和知情同意。
2. 首选诊断性放疗的适应证为：临床及影像学支持生殖细胞瘤的诊断，无严重颅高压症状，肿瘤标志物检查不支持绒毛膜上皮癌、胚胎癌、内胚窦瘤（卵黄囊瘤）；放疗1周左右复查脑MRI，如肿瘤缩小，继续放疗，否则停止。
3. 诊断性化疗治疗1周期后复查脑MRI，如肿瘤缩小，继续化疗，否则停止。

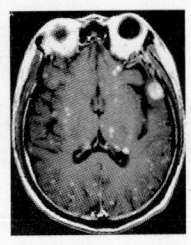

第七章
脑转移瘤

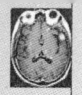

脑转移瘤

在成人中，脑转移瘤是最常见的颅内肿瘤，比原发脑肿瘤发病率高 10 倍左右。20%～40%的恶性肿瘤患者会出现脑转移。近几年，脑转移瘤的发病率有增高的趋势，可能与肿瘤发病率的增高、肿瘤患者生存时间延长、检查手段的进步有关。脑转移瘤最常见的原发灶有：肺癌、乳腺癌、结直肠癌、恶性黑色素瘤，其中来源于肺的约占一半。脑转移瘤中多发转移约占 70%～80%。脑转移瘤好发在脑灰白质交界处，因该部位血管管径相对狭窄，癌栓容易滞留。80%的脑转移在大脑半球，15%在小脑，5%在脑干。脑转移瘤的临床表现主要有两大类：颅内高压症状及局部症状。标准的影像学检查为颅脑 MRI 平扫加增强，其敏感性及解剖分辨率显著优于 CT。对于颅内病变与原发肿瘤关系不肯定者，强烈推荐行颅内病变立体定向活检或切除活检。

脑转移瘤的治疗目前仍没有统一的治疗模式可循，但各种治疗手段的选择时应结合患者的具体情况综合考虑。原发肿瘤的情况和处理会影响脑转移灶的处理考虑。目前的治疗手段包括全脑放疗（whole brain radiotherapy，WBRT）和立体定向放疗（stereotactic radiosurgery，SRS）、手术治疗、化疗和对症支持治疗。

2010 年 1 月，AANS 联合 CNS 制定公布了脑转移瘤的治疗指南。该指南是在 1990—2008 年 16 966 篇相关文献的基础上按照循证医学标准制定的，对脑转移瘤的不同治疗方式提出了规范性建议。

1. 对于初诊、单一脑转移灶、颅外病灶较局限、一般情况好可接受手术治疗的患者，Ⅰ级证据显示，手术联合术后

WBRT 能够提高颅内局控率,效果优于单纯手术或单纯 WBRT。但原发癌为相对放射敏感肿瘤,如小细胞肺癌、白血病、淋巴瘤、生殖细胞瘤及多发性骨髓瘤除外。

2. 对于初诊脑转移瘤患者,Ⅰ级证据显示,改变全脑放疗的分割方式并未能改善患者的中位生存时间、局部控制率及认知能力的改善。且目前暂无证据支持可根据不同的组织病理类型选择不同的剂量分割方式。

3. 对于初诊、单一脑转移灶、可接受手术治疗的患者,Ⅱ级证据显示,手术+WBRT 与 SRS+WBRT 比较,两者在改善患者生存率上无明显差异。但在肿块>3cm 或占位效应较明显(中线偏移>1cm)患者中,并无证据支持 SRS 可获益。

4. 对于肿块最大径<3cm 或者占位效应不明显(中线偏移小于 1cm)的患者:

①Ⅰ级证据显示,KPS≥70 分者,SRS+WBRT 优于 WBRT,可延长患者生存时间。Ⅰ级证据显示,对于 KPS 评分≥70 分且存在 1~4 个脑转移瘤的患者,SRS+WBRT 在肿瘤局部控制和功能维持方面比单纯 WBRT 更有优势。Ⅱ级证据显示,对于存在 2~3 个脑转移瘤的患者,与单纯 WBRT 相比,SRS+WBRT 能够显著延长生存时间。Ⅲ级证据显示,对于 KPS 评分<70 分且存在单个或多个脑转移瘤的患者,SRS+WBRT 比单纯 WBRT 能够提高患者的生存率。

②Ⅱ级证据显示,SRS+WBRT 与单纯 SRS 疗效比较,单纯 SRS 治疗脑转移瘤能够获得与 SRS+WBRT 相近的生存率。

③Ⅱ级证据显示,外科手术切除+WBRT 与 SRS±WBRT 疗效比较,两种方法疗效相近。

④Ⅲ级证据显示,SRS 与 WBRT 疗效比较,虽然两种方法单独应用均有良好效果,但 SRS 更能使存在 3 个以上脑转

移瘤的患者的生存获益。

5. 对于初诊的脑转移瘤，但不包括化疗敏感的原发肿瘤脑转移，如生殖细胞瘤脑转移：Ⅰ级证据显示，WBRT后常规化疗并未能使患者生存获益，故不推荐。4个Ⅰ级研究结果显示卡铂、氯乙基亚硝基脲类、喃氟啶、替莫唑胺等化疗药均未能使患者生存获益。但是由于这些数据多数来源于原发灶为非小细胞肺癌及乳腺癌，而且在某些临床试验中显示化疗＋WBRT可提高反应率，故临床医师应根据不同患者做个体化选择，并鼓励患者参加与化疗有关的临床试验。

6. 对于复发或脑转移进展的患者，应根据患者的以下几种情况做出治疗选择：患者的功能状态、肿瘤的广泛程度、脑转移灶的个数及体积、是否原脑转移部位复发或转移、之前的治疗手段以及原发瘤的病理类型等。治疗手段有：最佳支持治疗、再次放疗（WBRT或SRS）、手术切除或化疗。

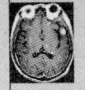

第七章 脑转移瘤

脑转移瘤（1~3个转移灶）诊疗流程

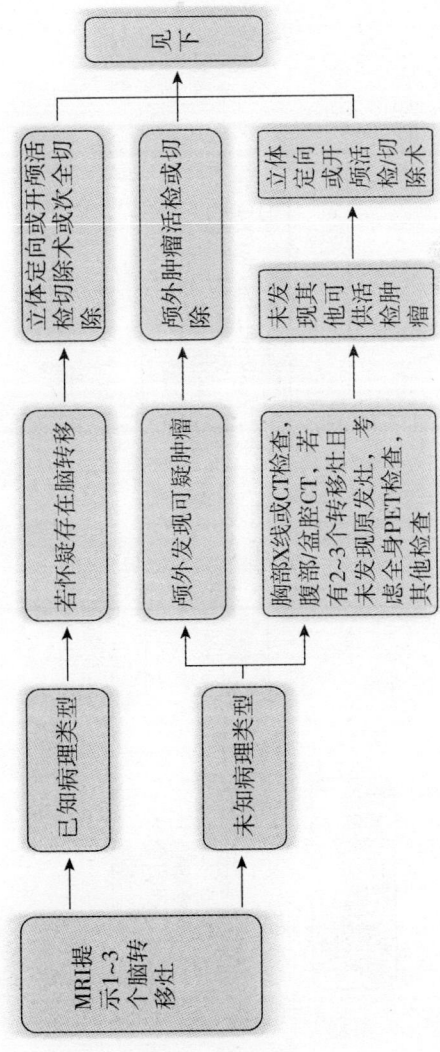

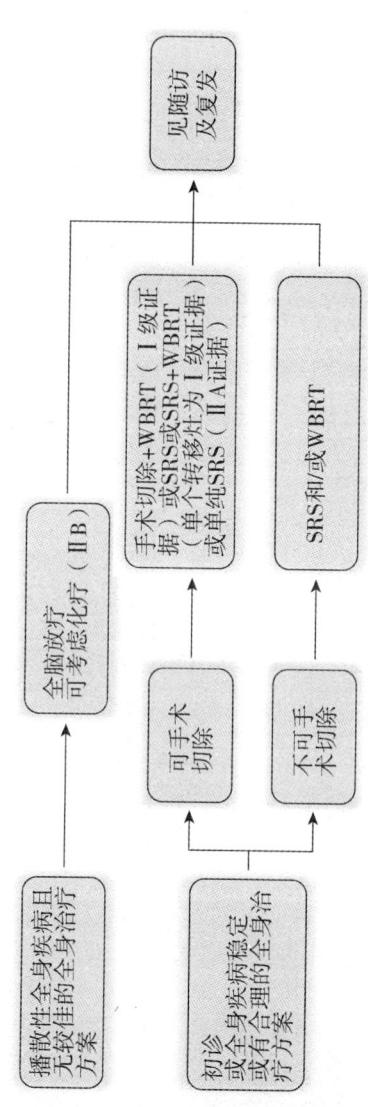

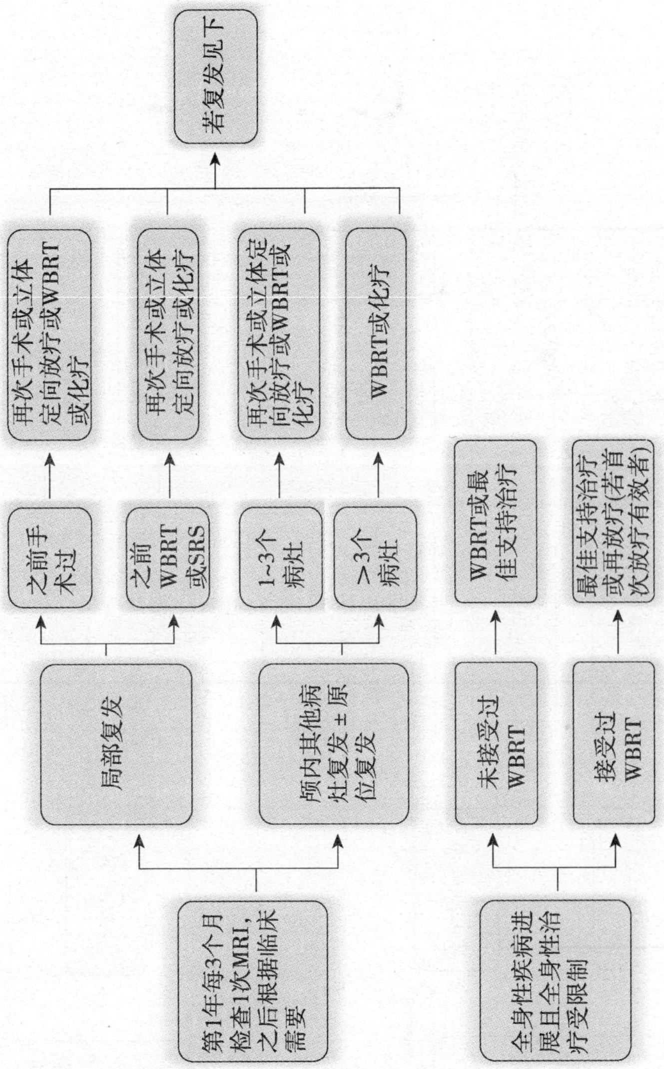

第七章 脑转移瘤

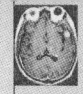

```
第1年每3个月           ┌─ 局部复发 ──┬─ 之前手术过 ──────→ 再次手术或立体定向放疗或WBRT或化疗 ─┐
检查1次MRI,            │            └─ 之前WBRT或SRS ──→ 再次手术或立体定向放疗或化疗 ──────┤
之后根据临床 ──────────┤                                                                  ├──→ 若复发见下
需要                   └─ 颅内其他病灶复发±原位复发 ──┬─ 1~3个病灶 ──→ 再次手术或立体定向放疗或WBRT或化疗 ─┤
                                                     └─ >3个病灶 ───→ WBRT或化疗 ─────────┘

全身性疾病进 ──────────┬─ 未接受过WBRT ──→ WBRT或最佳支持治疗
展且全身性治             │
疗受限制               └─ 接受过WBRT ───→ 最佳支持治疗或再放疗(对首次放疗有效者)
```

脑转移瘤（3个以上转移灶）诊疗流程

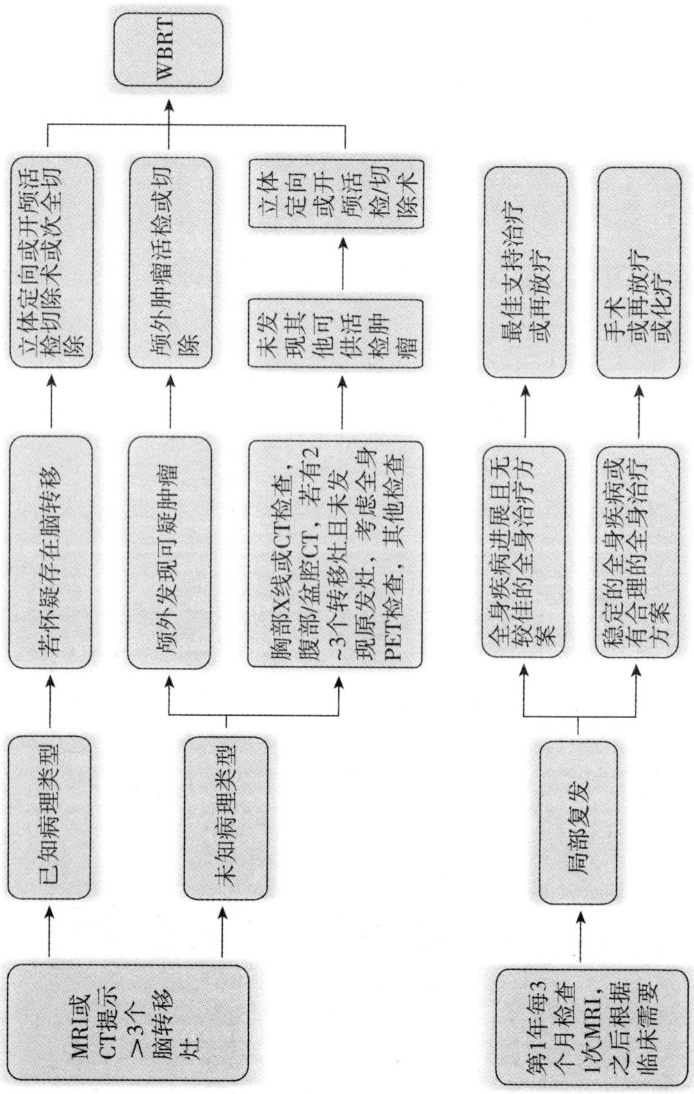

```
MRI或CT提示>3个脑转移灶
├── 已知病理类型
│   └── 若怀疑存在脑转移
│       └── 立体定向或开颅活检切除术或改全切除 → WBRT
└── 未知病理类型
    ├── 颅外发现可疑肿瘤
    │   └── 颅外肿瘤活检或切除 → WBRT
    └── 胸部X线或CT检查，腹腔/盆腔CT，若有2~3个转移灶且未发现原发灶，考虑全身PET检查，其他检查
        ├── 未发现其他可供活检肿瘤
        │   └── 立体定向或开颅活检切除术 → WBRT
        
第1年每3个月检查1次MRI，之后根据临床需要
└── 局部复发
    ├── 全身疾病进展且无较佳的全身治疗方案 → 最佳支持治疗或再放疗
    └── 稳定的全身疾病或有合理的全身治疗方案 → 手术或再放疗或化疗
```

第八章

神经系统肿瘤常用化疗方案

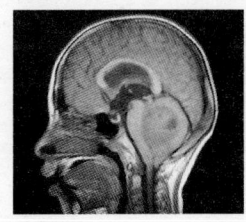

恶性胶质瘤

方案	药物	剂量	给药途径	给药时间	周期
CCNU+PCZ+VCR	CCNU	110mg/m²	PO	D1	6周
	PCZ	60mg/(m²·d)	PO	D8-21	
	VCR	1.4mg/(m²·d) (max 2mg)	IV	D8,29	
BCNU+DDP	BCNU	40mg/(m²·d)	IV	D1-3	4周
	DDP	40mg/(m²·d)	IV	D1-3	
MeCCNU+VM-26	MeCCNU	125mg/m²	PO	D3	6周
	VM-26	100mg/(m²·d)	IV	D1-3	
ACNU+VM-26	ACNU	90 mg/m²	IV	D1	6周
	VM-26	60mg/(m²·d)	IV	D1-3	
TMZ同步放疗	TMZ	75 mg/(m²·d)	PO	D1-42	放疗期间同步
TMZ 5/28d	TMZ	150~200mg/(m²·d)	PO	D1-5	4周
TMZ 21/28d	TMZ	75~100 mg/(m²·d)	PO	D1-21	4周
TMZ 7d/7d	TMZ	150 mg/(m²·d)	PO	D1-7,15-21	4周
TMZ daily	TMZ	50 mg/(m²·d)	PO	D1-28	4周
TMZ+DDP	TMZ	150~200 mg/(m²·d)	PO	D2-6	4周
	DDP	40mg/(m²·d)	IV	D1,2	
TMZ+VM-26	TMZ	150~200mg/(m²·d)	PO	D1-5	4周
	VM-26	100mg/(m²·d)	IV	D1-3	
TMZ+CPT-11	TMZ	200mg/(m²·d)	PO	D1-5	4周
	CPT-11	125mg/(m²·d)	IV	D6,13,20	

续表

方案	药物	剂量	给药途径	给药时间	周期
TMZ+PCB	TMZ	200mg/(m²·d)	PO	D1-5	4周
	PCB	100mg/(m²·d)，TMZ前1h	PO	D1-5	
VM-26+DDP	VM-26	100mg/(m²·d)	IV	D1-3	3~4周
	DDP	80mg/m²	IV	D1	
VM-26+CBP	VM-26	100mg/(m²·d)	IV	D1-3	3~4周
	CBP	300mg/m²	IV	D1	
Bevacizumab±CPT-11	Bevacizumab	10mg/kg	IV	D1,15	4周
	CPT-11	125mg/m²(non-EIAEDs)或340 mg/m²(EIAEDs)	IV	D1,15	
Bevacizumab±TMZ	Bevacizumab	10mg/kg	IV	D1,15	4周
	TMZ	50 mg/(m²·d)	PO	D1-28	

髓母细胞瘤

方案	药物	剂量	给药途径	给药时间	周期
CCNU+DDP+VCR	CCNU	75mg/m²	PO	D1	6周
	DDP	60~75mg/m²	IV	D1	
	VCR	1.4mg/(m²·d) (max 2mg)	IV	D1,8,15	
CCNU+Pred+VCR	CCNU	100mg/m²	PO	D1	6周
	Prednisone	40mg/(m²·d)	PO	D1-14	
	VCR	1.4mg/(m²·d) (max 2mg)	IV	D1,8,15	

续表

方案	药物	剂量	给药途径	给药时间	周期
VP-16+CBP	VP-16	80~100mg/(m^2·d)	IV	D1-4	3周
	CBP	300~400mg/m^2	IV	D1	
IFO+CBP+VP-16	IFO	2000mg/(m^2·d)(mesna 解毒)	IV	D1-3	4周
	CBP	400mg/m^2	IV	D1	
	VP-16	100mg/(m^2·d)	IV	D1-3	

原发性中枢神经系统生殖细胞肿瘤

方案	药物	剂量	给药途径	给药时间	周期
PEB	DDP	100mg/m^2	IV	D1	3~4周
	VM-26/VP-16	80mg/(m^2·d)	IV	D1-5	
	BLM	10mg/(m^2·d)	IV	D1, 5	

原发性中枢神经系统淋巴瘤

方案	药物	剂量	给药途径	给药时间	周期
HD-MTX	MTX	≥3000mg/m^2	IV	D1	3周

（注：注意检测 MTX 血药浓度，CF 解救，碱化、水化；由于毒性大，在有条件的医院才能实施）

第九章

神经系统肿瘤常用放疗方案

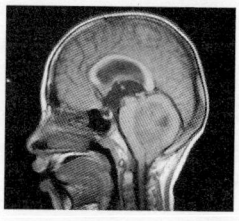

高级别星形细胞肿瘤

靶区：

GTV1 = T1 加权增强 + T2 加权/FLAIR，CTV1 = GTV1 + 外放 2 cm

GTV2 = T1 加权增强，CTV2 = GTV2 + 外放 2 cm

PTV = CTV + 外放 0.5 cm

分割剂量：1.8～2.2 Gy/次，每周 5 次

处方剂量：GTV1 = 46～50 Gy；GTV2 = 60～66 Gy

低级别星形细胞肿瘤

靶区：

GTV = T1 加权增强或 FLAIR 的异常区域

CTV = GTV + 外放 1～2 cm

PTV = CTV + 外放 0.5 cm

分割剂量：2.0 Gy/次，每周 5 次

处方剂量：GTV 46～60 Gy

室管膜瘤

(1) CSF 阴性

靶区：

GTV = T1 加权增强或 T2 加权/FLAIR 的异常区域

CTV = GTV + 外放 1~2 cm

PTV = CTV + 外放 0.5 cm

分割剂量：1.8~2.0 Gy/次，每周 5 次

处方剂量：GTV 56~60 Gy

(2) CSF 阳性

靶区：

GTV1 = T1 加权增强 + T2 加权/FLAIR，CTV1 = GTV1 + 外放 2 cm

GTV2 = T1 加权增强，CTV2 = GTV2 + 外放 2 cm

PTV = CTV + 外放 0.5 cm

分割剂量：1.8~2.2 Gy/次，每周 5 次

处方剂量：GTV1 = 46~50 Gy；GTV2 = 60~66 Gy

髓母细胞瘤

(1) 非高危病人：年龄大于 3 岁，残留病灶小于 $1.5 cm^2$，没有远处转移

GTV = MRI 的异常区域

CTV1 = 全中枢

CTV2 = GTV + 外放 2 cm + 颅后窝

PTV = CTV + 外放 0.5 cm

分割剂量：1.8 Gy/次，每周 5 次

处方剂量：CTV1 = 23.4 Gy；CTV2 = 54 Gy

(2) 高危病人：年龄小于 3 岁，或残留病灶大于 $1.5 cm^2$，或有远处转移

GTV = MRI 的异常区域

CTV1 = 全中枢

CTV2 = GTV + 外放 2 cm + 后颅窝

PTV = CTV + 外放 0.5 cm

分割剂量：1.8 Gy/次，每周 5 次

处方剂量：CTV1 = 36～39 Gy；CTV2 = 54 Gy

中枢神经系统淋巴瘤

(1) 单纯放疗

靶区：

GTV = T1 加权增强 + T2 加权/FLAIR

CTV1 = 全脑

CTV2 = GTV + 外放 2 cm

PTV = CTV + 外放 0.5 cm

分割剂量：1.8～2.0 Gy/次，每周 5 次

处方剂量：CTV1 = 40Gy；GTV = 60 Gy

(2) 化疗后辅助放疗

靶区：

GTV1 = T1 加权增强 + T2 加权/FLAIR，CTV1 = GTV1 + 外放 2 cm

GTV2（追加剂量）= T1 加权增强，CTV2 = GTV2 + 外放 2 cm

PTV = CTV + 外放 0.5 cm

分割剂量：1.8～2.2 Gy/次，每周 5 次

处方剂量：GTV1 = 26～36 Gy；GTV2 = 36～50Gy

原发性中枢神经系统生殖细胞肿瘤

(1) 生殖细胞瘤

单纯松果体区侵犯

靶区：

GTV = MRI 的异常区域

CTV1 = GTV + 外放 2 cm + 全脑室

CTV2 = GTV + 外放 2 cm

PTV = CTV + 外放 0.5 cm

分割剂量：1.8~2.0 Gy/次，每周 5 次

处方剂量：CTV1 = 30 Gy；GTV = 50 Gy

松果体外中枢神经系统侵犯

靶区：

GTV = MRI 的异常区域

CTV1 = 中枢神经系统

CTV2 = GTV + 外放 2 cm

PTV = CTV + 外放 0.5 cm

分割剂量：1.8~2.0 Gy/次，每周 5 次

处方剂量：CTV1 = 30~36 Gy；GTV = 50 Gy

（2）NGGT

单纯松果体区侵犯

靶区：

GTV = MRI 的异常区域

CTV = GTV + 外放 2 cm

PTV = CTV + 外放 0.5 cm

分割剂量：1.8~2.0 Gy/次，每周 5 次

处方剂量：GTV = 50 Gy

松果体外中枢神经系统侵犯

靶区：

GTV = MRI 的异常区域

CTV1 = 中枢神经系统

CTV2 = GTV + 外放 2 cm

PTV = CTV + 外放 0.5 cm

分割剂量：1.8~2.0 Gy/次，每周 5 次

处方剂量：CTV1 = 30~36 Gy；GTV = 50 Gy

附录一

纲要参考的循证医学依据级别

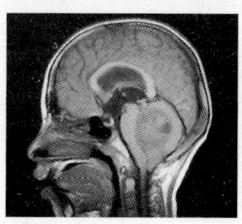

纲要参考的循证医学依据级别

等级	循证医学依据
I	高质量的循证依据（对随机对照临床试验（RCT）的 Meta 分析结果或大样本多中心 RCT 结果）
IIA	非高质量的循证依据，但结果一致
IIB	非高质量的循证依据，而且结果不一致（但没有大的不同）
III	任何等级的循证依据，而且结果存在大的不同

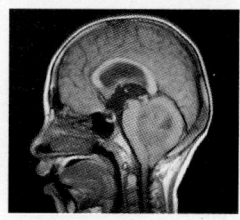

附录二
英文缩略语表

英文缩略语表

英文缩写	英文全称	中文释义
AA	anaplastic astrocytoma	间变性星形细胞瘤
AO	anaplastic oligodendroglioma	间变性少突胶质细胞瘤
AOA	anaplastic oligodendro-astrocytoma	间变性少突-星形细胞瘤
CNS	central nervous system	中枢神经系统
GBM	glioblastoma	胶质母细胞瘤
GCTs	germ cell tumors	生殖细胞肿瘤
KPS	Karnofsky Performance Scale	卡诺夫斯基健康状况量表
LI	labeling index	增殖指数
PNETs	primitive neuroectodermal tumours	原始神经外胚层肿瘤
PCNSL	primary central nervous system lymphoma	原发性中枢神经系统淋巴瘤
WBRT	whole brain radiotherapy	全脑放疗
SRS	stereotactic radiosurgery	立体定向放疗

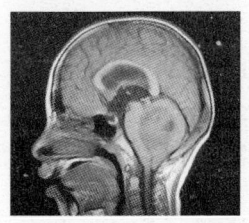

附录三
参考文献

胶质瘤

1. Sawaya R, Hammoud M, Schoppa D, et al. Neurosurgical outcomes in a modern series of 400 craniotomies for treatment of parenchymal tumors. Neurosurgery, 1998, 42:1044 – 1055.
2. Curran WJ, Scott CB, Horton J, et al. Recursive partitioning analysis of prognostic factors in three Radiation Therapy Oncology Group malignant glioma trials. J Natl Cancer Inst, 1993, 85:704 – 710.
3. Laws ER, Parney IF, Huang W, et al. Survival following surgery and prognostic factors for recently diagnosed malignant glioma: data from the Glioma Outcomes Project. J Neurosurg, 2003, 99:467 – 473.
4. Hentschel SJ, Sawaya R. Optimizing outcomes with maximal surgical resection of malignant gliomas. Cancer Control, 2003, 10:109 – 114.
5. Harsh GR 4th, Levin VA, Gutin PH, et al. Reoperation for recurrent glioblastoma and anaplastic astrocytoma. Neurosurgery, 1987, 21:615 – 621.
6. Roa W, Brasher PM, Bauman G, et al. Abbreviated course of radiation therapy in older patients with glioblastoma multiforme: a prospective randomized clinical trial. J Clin Oncol, 2004, 22:1583 – 1588.
7. Souhami L, Seiferheld W, Brachman D, et al. Randomized comparison of stereotactic radiosurgery followed by conventional radiotherapy with carmustine to conventional radiotherapy with carmustine for patients with glioblastoma multiforme: report of Radiation Therapy Oncology Group 93 – 05 protocol. Int J Radiat Oncol Biol Phys, 2004, 60:853 – 860.
8. Laperriere NJ, Leung PM, McKenzie S, et al. Randomized study of brachytherapy in the initial management of patients with malignant astrocytoma. Int J Radiat Oncol Biol Phys, 1998, 41:1005 – 1011.
9. Medical Research Council Brain Tumor Working Party. Randomized

trial of procarbazine, lomustine, and vincristine in the adjuvant treatment of high-grade astrocytoma: a Medical Research Council trial. J Clin Oncol, 2001, 19:509-518.

10. Fine HA, Dear BG, Loeffler JS, et al. Meta-analysis of radiation therapy with and without adjuvant chemotherapy for malignant gliomas in adults. Cancer, 1993, 71: 2585-2597.

11. Glioma Meta-analysis Trialists (GMT) Group. Chemotherapy for high-grade glioma. Cochrane Database Syst Rev, 2002, (4):CD003913.

12. Stupp R, Mason WP, van den Bent MJ, et al. Radiotherapy plus concomitant and adjuvant temozolomide for glioblastoma. N Engl J Med, 2005, 352:987-996.

13. Hegi ME, Diserens AC, Gorlia T, et al. MGMT gene silencing and benefit from temozolomide in glioblastoma. N Engl J Med, 2005, 352:997-1003.

14. Mollemann M, Wolter M, Felsberg J, et al. Frequent promoter hypermethylation and low expression of the MGMT gene in oligodendroglial tumors. Int J Cancer, 2005, 113:379-385.

15. Glantz M, Chamberlain MC, Liu Q, et al. Temozolomide as an alternative to irradiation for elderly patients with newly diagnosed malignant gliomas. Cancer, 2003, 97:2262-2266.

16. Brandes AA, Vastola F, Basso U, et al. A prospective study on glioblastoma in the elderly. Cancer, 2003, 97:657-662.

17. Levin VA, Silva P, Hannigan J, et al. Superiority of postradiotherapy adjuvant chemotherapy with CCNU, procarbazine and vincristine (PCV) over BCNU for anaplastic glioma: NCOG 6G61 final report. Int J Radiat Oncol Biol Phys, 1990, 18:321-324.

18. Prados MD, Scott C, Curran WJ Jr, et al. Procarbazine, lomustine, and vincristine (PCV) chemotherapy for anaplastic astrocytoma: A retrospective review of radiation therapy oncology group protocols comparing survival with carmustine or PCV adjuvant chemotherapy. J Clin Oncol, 1999, 17:3389-3395.

19. Brandes AA, Tosoni A, Basso U, et al. Second-line chemotherapy

with irinotecan plus carmustine in glioblastoma recurrent or progressive after first-line temozolomide chemotherapy: a phase II study of the Gruppo Italiano Cooperativo di Neuro – Oncologia (GICNO). J Clin Oncol, 2004, 22:4779–4786.
20. Reardon DA, Quinn JA, Vredenburgh J, et al. Phase II trial of irinotecan plus celecoxib in adults with recurrent malignant glioma. Cancer, 2005, 103:329–338.
21. Brandes AA, Basso U, Reni M, et al. First-line chemotherapy with cisplatin plus fractionated temozolomide in recurrent glioblastoma multiforme: A phase II study of the Gruppo Italiano Cooperativo di Neuro-Oncologia. J Clin Oncol, 2004, 22: 1598–1604.
22. Vredenburgh JJ, Desjardins A, Herndon JE, II, et al. Bevacizumab plus irinotecan in recurrent glioblastoma multiforme. J Clin Oncol, 2007, 25:4722–4729.
23. Crews KR, Stewart CF, Jones-Wallace D, et al. Altered irinotecan pharmacokinetics in pediatric high-grade glioma patients receiving enzyme-inducing anticonvulsant therapy. Clin Cancer Res, 2002, 8:2202–2209.
24. Vecht CJ, Wagner GL, Wilms EB. Interactions between antiepileptic and chemotherapeutic drugs. Lancet Neurol, 2003, 2:404–409.
25. Gilbert MR, Supko JG, Batchelor T, et al. Phase I clinical and pharmacokinetic study of irinotecan in adults with recurrent malignant glioma. Clin Cancer Res, 2003, 9:2940–2949.
26. Cairncross G, Berkey B, Shaw E, et al. Phase III trial of chemotherapy plus radiotherapy compared with radiotherapy alone for pure and mixed anaplastic oligodendroglioma: Intergroup Radiation Therapy Oncology Group Trial 9402. J Clin Oncol, 2006, 24:2707–2714.
27. van den Bent MJ, Carpentier AF, Brandes AA, et al. Adjuvant procarbazine, lomustine, and vincristine improves progression-free survival but not overall survival in newly diagnosed anaplastic oligodendrogliomas and oligoastrocytomas: a randomized European Organisation for Research and Treatment of Cancer phase III trial. J Clin Oncol, 2006, 24:2715–2722.

28. Yung WK, Prados MD, Yaya-Tur R, et al. Multicenter phase II trial of temozolomide in patients with anaplastic astrocytoma or anaplastic oligoastrocytoma at first relapse: Temodal Brain Tumor Group. J Clin Oncol, 1999,17:2672-2771.
29. van den Bent MJ, Taphoorn MJ, Brandes AA, et al. Phase II study of first-line chemotherapy with temozolomide in recurrent oligodendroglial tumors: the European Organization for Research and Treatment of Cancer Brain Tumor Group Study 26791. J Clin Oncol, 2003,21:2525-2528.
30. Silvani A, Eoli M, Salmaggi A, et al. Phase II trial of cisplatin plus temozolomide, in recurrent and progressive malignant glioma patients. J Neurooncol,2004,66: 203-208.
31. Wick A, Felsberg J, Steinbach JP, et al. Efficacy and tolerability of temozolomide in an alternating weekly regimen in patients with recurrent glioma. J Clin Oncol,2007, 25:3357-3361.
32. Shaw EG, Daumas-Duport C, Scheithauer BW, et al. Radiation therapy in the management of low-grade supratentorial astrocytomas. J Neurosurg,1989,70:853-861.
33. Keles GE, Lamborn KR, Berger MS. Low-grade hemispheric gliomas in adults: a critical review of extent of resection as a factor influencing outcome. J Neurosurg, 2001,95:735-745.
34. Soffietti R, Chio A, Giordana MT, et al. Prognostic factors in well differentiated cerebral astrocytomas in the adult. Neurosurg, 1989,26:686-692.
35. Philippon JH, Clemenceau SH, Fauchon FH, et al. Supratentorial low-grade astrocytomas in adults. Neurosurg, 1993,32:554-559.
36. Lo SS, Cho KH, Hall WA, et al. Does the extent of surgery have an impact on the survival of patients who receive postoperative radiation therapy for supratentorial low-grade gliomas? Int J Cancer, 2001,96 (Suppl):71-78.
37. Kilic T, Ozduman K, Elmaci I, et al. Effect of surgery on tumor progression and malignant degeneration in hemispheric diffuse low grade astrocytomas. J Clin Neurosci, 2002,9:549-552.

38. Berger MS, Deliganis AVK, Dobbins J, et al. The effect of extent of resection on recurrence in patients with low grade cerebral hemisphere gliomas. Cancer, 1994, 74: 1784-1791.
39. Karim AB, Afra D, Cornu P, et al. Randomized trial on the efficacy of radiotherapy for cerebral low-grade glioma in the adult: European Organization for Research and Treatment of Cancer Study 22845 with the Medical Research Council study BRO4: an interim analysis. Int J Radiat Oncol Biol Phys, 2002, 52:316-324.
40. van den Bent MJ, Afra D, de Witte O, et al. Long-term efficacy of early versus delayed radiotherapy for low-grade astrocytoma and oligodendroglioma in adults: the EORTC 22845 randomised trial. Lancet, 2005, 366:985-990.
41. Shaw EG, Tatter SB, Lesser GJ, et al. Current controversies in the radiotherapeutic management of adult low-grade glioma. Semin Oncol, 2004, 31: 653-658.
42. Shaw EG, Wisoff JH. Prospective clinical trials of intracranial low grade glioma in adults and children. Neuro Oncol, 2003, 5:153-160.
43. Karim AB, Maat B, Hatlevoll R, et al. A randomized trial on doseresponse in radiation therapy of low-grade cerebral glioma: European Organization for Research and Treatment of Cancer (EORTC) study 22844. Int J Radiat Oncol Biol Phys, 1996, 36: 549-556.
44. Shaw E, Arusell R, Scheithauer B, et al. Prospective randomized trial of low-versus high-dose radiation therapy in adults with supratentorial low-grade glioma: Initial report of a North Central Cancer Treatment Group/Radiation Therapy Oncology Group/Eastern Cooperative Oncology Group study. J Clin Oncol, 2002, 20:2267-2276.
45. Quinn JA, Reardon DA, Friedman AH, et al. Phase II trial of temozolomide in patients with progressive low-grade glioma. J Clin Oncol, 2003, 21:646-651.
46. Lo SS, Hall WA, Cho KH, et al. Radiation dose response for supratentorial low-grade glioma-institutional experience and literature

review. J Neurol Sci, 2003, 214:43 - 48.
47. Nijjar TS, Simpson WJ, Gadalla T, et al. Oligodendroglioma: The Princess Margaret Hospital experience (1958 - 1984). Cancer, 1993, 71:4002 - 4006.
48. Cairncross JG, Ueki K, Zlatescu M, et al. Specific genetic predictors of chemotherapeutic response and survival in patients with anaplastic oligodendrogliomas. J Natl Cancer Inst, 1998, 90:1473 - 1479.
49. Lindegaard KF, Mork SJ, Eide GE, et al. Statistical analysis of clinicopathological features, radiotherapy, and survival in 170 cases of oligodendroglioma. J Neurosurg, 1987, 67:224 - 230.
50. Shaw EG, Scheithauer BW, O'Fallon JR, et al. Mixed oligoastrocytomas: A survival and prognostic factor analysis. Neurosurg, 1994, 34:577 - 582.
51. Shaw EG, Scheithauer BW, O'Fallon JR, et al. Oligodendrogliomas: The Mayo Clinic experience. J Neurosurg, 1992, 76:428 - 434.
52. Mork SJ, Lindegaard KF, Halvorsen TB, et al. Oligodendroglioma: Incidence and biological behaviour in a defined population. J Neurosurg, 1985, 63:881 - 889.
53. Yeh SA, Lee TC, Chen HJ, et al. Treatment outcomes and prognostic factors of patients with supratentorial low-grade oligodendroglioma. Int J Radiat Oncol Biol Phys, 2002, 54:1405 - 1409.
54. Cairncross G, Macdonald D, Ludwin S, et al. Chemotherapy for anaplastic oligodendroglioma. J Clin Oncol, 1994, 12:2013 - 2021.
55. Buckner JC, Gesme D Jr, O'Fallon JR, et al. Phase II trial of procarbazine, lomustine, and vincristine as initial therapy for patients with low-grade oligodendroglioma or oligoastrocytoma: efficacy and associations with chromosomal abnormalities. J Clin Oncol, 2003, 21:251 - 255.
56. van den Bent M, Chinot OL, Cairncross JG. Recent developments in the molecular characterization and treatment of oligodendroglial tumors. Neuro-oncol, 2003, 5:128 - 138.
57. Ino Y, Betensky RA, Zlatescu MC, et al. Molecular subtypes of anaplastic oligodendroglioma: implications for patient management

at diagnosis. Clin Cancer Res, 2001, 7: 839 - 845.
58. Berger MS, Rostomily RC. Low grade gliomas: Functional mapping resection strategies, extent of resection and outcome. J Neurooncol, 1997, 34: 85 - 101.
59. Buatti JM, Meeks SL, Ryken TC, et al. Low-grade gliomas: answering one question in a myriad of new questions [editorial]. J Clin Oncol, 2002, 20: 2223 - 2224.
60. Smith JS, Perry A, Borell TJ, et al. Alterations of chromosome arms 1p and 19q as predictors of survival in oligodendrogliomas, astrocytomas, and mixed oligoastrocytomas. J Clin Oncol, 2000, 18: 636 - 645.
61. van den Bent MJ. New perspectives for the diagnosis and treatment of oligodendroglioma. Expert Rev Anticancer Ther, 2001, 1: 348 - 356.
62. van den Bent MJ. Advances in the biology and treatment of oligodendrogliomas. Curr Opin Neurol, 2004, 17: 675 - 680.
63. Chinot O, Honore S, Dufour H, et al. Safety and efficacy of temozolomide in patients with recurrent anaplastic oligodendrogliomas after standard radiotherapy and chemotherapy. J Clin Oncol, 2001, 19: 2449 - 2455.
64. Hoang-Xuan K, Capelle L, Kujas M, et al. Temozolomide as initial treatment for adults with low-grade oligodendrogliomas or oligoastrocytomas and correlation with chromosome 1p deletions. J Clin Oncol, 2004, 22: 3133 - 3138.
65. Vanuytsel LJ, Bessell EM, Ashley SE, et al. Intracranial ependymoma: Long-term results of a policy of surgery and radiotherapy. Int J Radiat Oncol Biol Phys, 1992, 23: 313 - 319.
66. Goldwein JW, Corn BW, Finlay JL, et al. Is craniospinal irradiation required to cure children with malignant (anaplastic) intracranial ependymomas? Cancer, 1991, 67: 2766 - 2771.
67. Wallner KE, Wara WM, Sheline GE, et al. Intracranial ependymomas: Results of treatment with partial or whole brain irradiation without spinal irradiation. Int J Radiat Oncol Biol Phys, 1986, 12: 1937 - 1941.
68. Vanuytsel L, Brada M. The role of prophylactic spinal irradiation

in localized intracranial ependymoma. Int J Radiat Oncol Biol Phys, 1991, 21: 825.

69. Mansur DB, Perry A, Rajaram V, et al. Postoperative radiation therapy for grade II and III intracranial ependymoma. Int J Radiat Oncol Biol Phys, 2005, 61: 387 – 391.

70. Wick A, Felsberg J, Steinbach JP, Herrlinger U, Platten M, Blaschke B, Meyermann R, Reifenberger G, Weller M, Wick W. Efficacy and tolerability of temozolomide in an alternating weekly regimen in patients with recurrent glioma. J Clin Oncol, 2007, 25 (22): 3357 – 3361.

71. Wolff JE, Berrak S, Koontz Webb SE, Zhang M. Nitrosourea efficacy in high-grade glioma: a survival gain analysis summarizing 504 cohorts with 24193 patients. J Neurooncol, 2008, 88(1): 57 – 63.

72. Albert FK, Forsting M, Sartor K, et al. Early postoperative magnetic resonance imaging after resection of malignant glioma: objective evaluation of residual tumor and its influence on regrowth and prognosis. Neurosurgery, 1994, 34(1): 45 – 60; discussion 41 – 60.

73. Stewart LA. Chemotherapy in adult high – grade glioma: a systematic review and meta-analysis of individual patient data from 12 randomised trials. Lancet, 2002, 359(9311): 1011 – 1018.

74. 李刚，牟永告，魏大年，张湘衡，杨群英，吴秋良，陈忠平. 替尼泊苷与尼莫司汀联合治疗 O6 -甲基鸟嘌呤- DNA 甲基转移酶（MGMT）阴性表达的恶性胶质细胞瘤：附 18 例经验. 中国神经肿瘤杂志，2009，7（1）：53 - 57.

75. 曾宪起，申长虹，浦佩玉，杨树源. 应用替莫唑胺对照司莫司丁治疗恶性脑胶质细胞瘤的疗效观察. 中华神经外科杂志，2006，22（4）：204 - 207.

76. 张俊平，牟永告，张湘衡，赛克，吴秋良，岳伟英，陈忠平. MGMT 表达指导下的恶性脑胶质细胞瘤预见性化疗近期疗效分析. 中华神经外科杂志，2007，23（2）：96 - 98.

77. 张俊平，赛克，魏大年，牟永告，张湘衡，吴秋良，陈忠平. MGMT 阳性恶性脑胶质细胞瘤病人的化疗（附 5 1 例体会）. 中华神经外科杂志，2007，23（9）：672 - 674.

髓母细胞瘤

1. Zeltzer PM, Boyett JM, Finlay JL, et al. Metastasis stage, adjuvant treatment, and residual tumor are prognostic factors for medulloblastoma in children:Conclusions from the Children's Cancer Group 921 randomized phase III study. J Clin Oncol, 1999, 17:832-845.
2. Thomas P, Deutsch M, Kepner JL, et al. Low stage medulloblastoma:Final analysis of trial comparing standard dose with reduced dose neuroaxis irradiation. J Clin Oncol, 2000, 18:3004-3011.
3. Bailey CC, Gnekow A, Wellek S, et al. Prospective randomized trial of chemotherapy given before radiotherapy in childhood medulloblastoma: International Society of Paediatric Oncology (SIOP) and the(German) Society of Paediatric Oncology(GPO):SIOP II. Med Pediatr Oncol,1995,25:166-178.
4. Kortmann RD, Kuhl J, Timmermann LA, et al. Post-operative neoadjuvant chemotherapy before radiotherapy as compared to immediate radiotherapy followed by maintenance chemotherapy in the treatment of medulloblastoma in childhood: Results of the German prospective randomized trial HIT 91. Int J Radiat Oncol Biol Phys, 2000,46:269-279.
5. Packer RJ, Goldwein J, Nicholson HS, et al. Treatment of children with medulloblastomas with reduced dose craniospinal radiation therapy and adjuvant chemotherapy: A Children's Cancer Group study. J Clin Oncol,1999,17:2127-2136.
6. Packer RJ, Gajjar A, Vezina G, et al. Phase III study of craniospinal radiation therapy followed by adjuvant chemotherapy for newly diagnosed average-risk medulloblastoma. J Clin Oncol, 2006, 25: 4202-4208.
7. Taylor RE, Bailey CC, Robinson KJ, et al. Outcome of patients with metastatic (M2-3) medulloblastoma treated with SIOP/UKCCSG

PNET-3 chemotherapy. Eur J Cancer, 2005, 41:727 - 734.
8. Jakacki RI, Zeltzer PM, Boyett JM, et al. Survival and prognostic factors following radiation and/or chemotherapy for primitive neuroectodermal tumom of the pineal region in infants and children: a report of the Childrens Cancer Group. J Clin Oncol, 1995, 13:1377 - 1383.
9. Gajjar A, Chintagnmpala M, Ashley D, et al. Risk-adapted craniospinal radiotherapy followed by high-dose chemotherapy and stem cell rescue in children with newly diagnosed medulloblastoma (St Jude Medulloblastoma-96): long-term results from a prospective, multicentre trial. Lancet Oncol, 2006, 7:813 - 820.
10. Dufner PK, Horowitz ME, Krischer JP, et al. Postoperative chemotherapy and delayed radiation in children less than three years of age with malignant brain tumom. N Engl J Med, 1993, 328:1725 - 1731.

原发性中枢神经系统生殖细胞肿瘤

1. Kleihues P, Louis DN, Scheithauer BW, et al. The WHO classification of tumors of the nervous system. J Neuropathol Exp Neurol, 2002, 61:215 - 225.
2. Matsutani M, Sano K, Takakura K, et al. Primary intracranial germ cell tumor: a clinical analysis of 153 histologically verified cases. J Neurosurg, 1997, 86:446 - 455.
3. Huh SJ, Shin KH, Kim IH, et al. Radiotherapy of intracranial germinomas. Radiother Oncol, 1996, 38:19 - 23.
4. Shirato H, Nishio M, Sawamura Y, et al. Analysis of long-term treatment of intracranial germinoma. Int J Radiat Oncol Biol Phys, 1997, 37:511 - 515.
5. Maity A, Shu HK, Janss A, et al. Craniospinal radiation in the treatment of biopsy-proven intracranial germinomas: twenty-five years experience in a single center. Int J Radiat Oncol Biol Phys,

2004,58:1165-1170.

6. Schoenfeld GO, Amdur RJ, Schmalfuss IM, et al. Low-dose prophylactic craniospinal radiotherapy for intracranial germinoma. Int J Radiat Oncol Biol Phys, 2006, 65:481-485.

7. Shikama N, Ogawa K, Tanaka S, et al. Lack of benefit of spinal irradiation in the primary treatment of intracranial germinoma: a multiinstitutional, retrospective view of 180 patients. Cancer, 2005, 104:126-134.

8. Baranzelli MC, Patte C, Boufet E, et al. Nonmetastatic intracranial germinoma the experience of the French Society of Pediatric Oncology. Cancer, 1997, 80:1792-1797.

9. Cefalo G, Gianni MC, Lombardi F, et al. Intracranial germinoma: dose a cisplatinum-based chemotherapeutic regimen permit to avoid whole CNS irradiation. Med Ped Oncol, 1995, 25: 303.

10. Sawamura Y, Ikeda J, Shirato H, et al. Germ cell tumors of the central nervous system: Treatment consideration based on 111 cases and their long-term clnical outcomes. Eur J Cancer, 1998:34: 104-110.

11. Robertson PL, Darosso RC, Alen JC. Improved modality of intracranial non-germinoma germ cel tumors with multimodality therapy. J Neuro Oncol, 1997, 32:71-80.

12. Calaminus G, Bamberg M, Baranzeli MC, et al. Intracranial germ cel tumors: a comprehensive update of the European data. Neuropediatrics, 1994, 25:26-32.

13. Hasegawa T, Kondziolka D, Hadjipanayis CG, et al. Stereotactic radiosurgery for CNS nongerminomatous germ cel tumors. Pediatr Neurosurg, 2003, 38:329-333.

原发性中枢神经系统淋巴瘤

1. Fine HA, Mayer RJ. Primary central nervous system lymphoma.

Ann Intern Med, 1993, 119:1093 - 1104.
2. Deangelis LM. Current management of primary central nervous system lymphoma. Oncology, 1995, 9:63 - 71.
3. Cot TR, Manns A, Hardy CR, et al. Epidemiology of brain lymphoma among people with or without acquired immunodeficiency syndrome. J Natl Cancer Inst, 1996, 88:675 - 679.
4. Johnson BA, Fram EK, Johnson PC, et al. The variable MR appearance of primary lymphoma of the central nervous system: Comparison with histopathologic features. Am J Neuroradiol, 1997, 18:563 - 572.
5. Deangelis LM. Cerebral lymphoma presenting as a nonenhancing lesion on computed tomographic/magnetic resonance scan. Ann Neurol, 1993, 33:308 - 311.
6. Abrey LE, Batchelor TT, Ferreri AJ, et al. International Primary CNS Lymphoma Collaborative Group: Report of an international workshop to standardize baseline evaluation and response criteria for primary CNS lymphoma. J Clin Oncol, 2005, 23:5034 - 5043.
7. Deangelis LM, Yahalom J, Heinemann MH, et al. Primary CNS lymphoma: Combined treatment with chemotherapy and radiotherapy. Neurology, 1990, 40:80 - 86.
8. Neuwelt EA, Goldman DL, Dahlborg SA, et al. Primary CNS lymphoma treated with osmotic blood-brain barrier disruption: Prolonged survival and preservation of cognitive function. J Clin Oncol, 1991, 9:1580 - 1590.
9. Nelson DF, Martz KL, Bonner H, et al. Non-Hodgkin's lymphoma of the brain: Can high dose, large volume radiation therapy improve survival? Report on a prospective trial by the Radiation Therapy Oncology Group (RTOG): RTOG 8315. Int J Radiat Oncol Biol Phys, 1992, 23:9 - 17.
10. Gavrilovic IT, Hormigo A, Yahalom J, et al. Long-term follow-up of high-dose methotrexate-based therapy with and without whole brain irradiation for newly diagnosed primary CNS lymphoma. J Clin Oncol, 2006, 24:4570 - 4574.

11. Gabbai AA, Hochberg FH, Linggood RM, et al. High-dose methotrexate for non-AIDS primary central nervous system lymphoma: Report of 13 cases. J Neurosurg, 1989, 70:190 - 194.
12. Hiraga S, Arita N, Ohnishi T, et al. Rapid infusion of high-dose methotrexate resulting in enhanced penetration into cerebrospinal fluid and intensified tumor response in primary central nervous system lymphomas. J Neurosurg, 1999, 91: 221 - 230.
13. Deangelis LM. Primary central nervous system lymphomas. Curr Treat Options Oncol, 2001, 2:309 - 318.
14. DeAngelis LM, Seiferheld W, Schold SC, et al. Combination chemotherapy and radiotherapy for primary central nervous system lymphoma: Radiation Therapy Oncology Group Study 93 - 10. J Clin Oncol, 2002, 20:4643 - 4648.
15. Freilich RJ, Delattre JY, Monjour A, et al. Chemotherapy without radiation therapy as initial treatment for primary CNS lymphoma in older patients. Neurology, 1996, 46:435 - 439.
16. Batchelor T, Carson K, O'Neill A, et al. Treatment of primary CNS lymphoma with methotrexate and deferred radiotherapy: a report of NABTT 96 - 07. J Clin Oncol, 2003, 21:1044 - 1049.
17. Nguyen PL, Chakravarti A, Finkelstein DM, et al. Results of whole brain radiation as salvage of methotrexate failure for immunocompetent patients with primary CNS lymphoma. J Clin Oncol, 2005, 23:1507 - 1513.
18. Wong ET, Tishler R, Barron L, et al. Immunochemotherapy with rituximab and temozolomide for central nervous system lymphomas. Cancer, 2004, 101:139 - 145.
19. Enting RH, Demopoulos A, Deangelis LM, et al. Salvage therapy for primary CNS lymphoma with a combination of rituximab and temozolomide. Neurology, 2004, 63:901 - 903.
20. Pitini V, Baldari S, Altavilla G, et al. Salvage therapy for primary central nervous system lymphoma with (90) Y-Ibritumomab and Temozolomide. Neurooncol, 2007, 83:291 - 293.
21. Voloschin AD, Betensky R, Wen PY, et al. Topotecan as salvage

therapy for relapsed or refractory primary central nervous system lymphoma. J Neurooncol, 2008,86:211-215.
22. Younes A, Preti HA, Hagemeister FB, et al. Paclitaxel plus topotecan treatment for patients with relapsed or refractory aggressive non-Hodgkin's lymphoma. Ann Oncol, 2001,12:923-927.
23. Martelli M, Vignetti M, Zinzani PL, et al. High-dose chemotherapy followed by autologous bone marrow transplantation versus dexamethasone, cisplatin, and cytarabine in aggressive non-Hodgkin's lymphoma with partial response to front-line chemotherapy: a prospective randomized Italian multicenter study. J Clin Oncol, 1996,14:534-542.

脑转移瘤

1. Barnholtz-Sloan JS, Sloan AE, Davis FG, et al. Incidence proportions of brain metastases in patients diagnosed (1973 to 2001) in the Metropolitan Detroit Cancer Surveillance System. J Clin Oncol, 2004,22:2865-2872.
2. Schouten LJ, Rutten J, Huveneers HA, Twijnstra A. Incidence of brain metastases in a cohort of patients with carcinoma of the breast, colon, kidney, and lung and melanoma. Cancer, 2002,94: 2698-2705.
3. Lin NU, Bellon JR, Winer EP. CNS metastases in breast cancer. J Clin Oncol, 2004, 22:3608-3617.
4. Eichler AF, Loeffler JS. Multidisciplinary management of brain metastases. Oncologist, 2007,12:884-898.
5. Barker FG, 2nd. Craniotomy for the resection of metastatic brain tumors in the U.S., 1988-2000: decreasing mortality and the effect of provider caseload. Cancer,2004,100:999-1007.
6. Patchell RA, Tibbs PA, Regine WF, et al. Postoperative radiotherapy in the treatment of single metastases to the brain: a ran-

domized trial. JAMA,1998,280:1485-1489.
7. Paek SH, Audu PB, Sperling MR, et al. Reevaluation of surgery for the treatment of brain metastases: review of 208 patients with single or multiple brain metastases treated at one institution with modern neurosurgical techniques. Neurosurgery, 2005, 56: 1021-1034.
8. Stark AM, Tscheslog H, Buhl R, et al. Surgical treatment for brain metastases: prognostic factors and survival in 177 patients. Neurosurg Rev,2005,28:115-119.
9. Suh JH. Stereotactic radiosurgery for the management of brain metastases. N Engl J Med, 2010,362:1119-1127.
10. Aoyama H, Shirato H, Tago M, et al. Stereotactic radiosurgery plus whole-brain radiation therapy vs stereotactic radiosurgery alone for treatment of brain metastases: a randomized controlled trial. JAMA, 2006,295:2483-2491.
11. O'Neill BP, Iturria NJ, Link MJ, et al. A comparison of surgical resection and stereotactic radiosurgery in the treatment of solitary brain metastases. Int J Radiat Oncol Biol Phys, 2003, 55: 1169-1176.
12. Rades D, Kueter JD, Veninga T, et al. Whole brain radiotherapy plus stereotactic radiosurgery (WBRT+SRS) versus surgery plus whole brain radiotherapy (OP+WBRT) for 1-3 brain metastases: results of a matched pair analysis. Eur J Cancer, 2009, 45: 400-404.
13. Schoggl A, Kitz K, Reddy M, et al. Defining the role of stereotactic radiosurgery versus microsurgery in the treatment of single brain metastases. Acta Neurochir (Wien), 2000, 142:621-626.
14. Muacevic A, Wowra B, Siefert A, et al. Microsurgery plus whole brain irradiation versus Gamma Knife surgery alone for treatment of single metastases to the brain: a randomized controlled multicentre phase III trial. J Neurooncol, 2008,87:299-307.
15. Akyurek S, Chang EL, Mahajan A, et al. Stereotactic radiosurgical treatment of cerebral metastases arising from breast cancer.

Am J Clin Oncol, 2007, 30:310 - 314.
16. Loeffler JS, Kooy HM, Wen PY, et al. The treatment of recurrent brain metastases with stereotactic radiosurgery. J Clin Oncol, 1990, 8:576 - 582.
17. Noel G, Medioni J, Valery CA, et al. Three irradiation treatment options including radiosurgery for brain metastases from primary lung cancer. Lung Cancer, 2003, 41:333 - 343.
18. Noel G, Proudhom MA, Valery CA, et al. Radiosurgery for reirradiation of brain metastasis: results in 54 patients. Radiother Oncol, 2001, 60:61 - 67.
19. Sheehan J, Kondziolka D, Flickinger J, Lunsford LD. Radiosurgery for patients with recurrent small cell lung carcinoma metastatic to the brain: outcomes and prognostic factors. J Neurosurg, 2005, 102 Suppl:247 - 254.
20. Patchell RA, Tibbs PA, Walsh JW, et al. A randomized trial of surgery in the treatment of single metastases to the brain. N Engl J Med, 1990, 322:494 - 500.
21. Vecht CJ, Haaxma-Reiche H, Noordijk EM, et al. Treatment of single brain metastasis: radiotherapy alone or combined with neurosurgery? Ann Neurol, 1993, 33:583 - 590.
22. Mintz AH, Kestle J, Rathbone MP, et al. A randomized trial to assess the efficacy of surgery in addition to radiotherapy in patients with a single cerebral metastasis. Cancer, 1996, 78:1470 - 1476.
23. Andrews DW, Scott CB, Sperduto PW, et al. Whole brain radiation therapy with or without stereotactic radiosurgery boost for patients with one to three brain metastases: phase III results of the RTOG 9508 randomised trial. Lancet, 2004, 363:1665 - 1672.
24. Kondziolka D, Patel A, Lunsford LD, et al. Stereotactic radiosurgery plus whole brain radiotherapy versus radiotherapy alone for patients with multiple brain metastases. Int J Radiat Oncol Biol Phys, 1999, 45:427 - 434.
25. Cooper JS, Steinfeld AD, Lerch IA. Cerebral metastases: value of reirradiation in selected patients. Radiology, 1990, 174:883 - 885.

26. Sadikov E, Bezjak A, Yi QL, et al. Value of whole brain reirradiation for brain metastases-single centre experience. Clin Oncol (R Coll Radiol), 2007,19:532-538.
27. Wong WW, Schild SE, Sawyer TE, Shaw EG. Analysis of outcome in patients reirradiated for brain metastases. Int J Radiat Oncol Biol Phys, 1996,34:585-590.
28. Guerrieri M, Wong K, Ryan G, et al. A randomised phase III study of palliative radiation with concomitant carboplatin for brain metastases from non-small cell carcinoma of the lung. Lung Cancer, 2004,46:107-111.
29. Verer E, Gil M, Yaya R, et al. Temozolomide and concomitant whole brain radiotherapy in patients with brain metastases: a phase II randomized trial. Int J Radiat Oncol Biol Phys, 2005,61:185-191.
30. Antonadou D, Paraskevaidis M, Sarris G, et al. Phase II randomized trial of temozolomide and concurrent radiotherapy in patients with brain metastases. J Clin Oncol, 2002,20:3644-3650
31. Agarwala SS, Kirkwood JM, Gore M, et al. Temozolomide for the treatment of brain metastases associated with metastatic melanoma: a phase II study. J Clin Oncol, 2004,22:2101-2107.
32. Krown SE, Niedzwiecki D, Hwu WJ, et al. Phase II study of temozolomide and thalidomide in patients with metastatic melanoma in the brain: high rate of thromboembolic events (CALGB 500102). Cancer, 2006,107:1883-1890.
33. Lassman AB, Abrey LE, Shah GD, et al. Systemic high-dose intravenous methotrexate for central nervous system metastases. J Neurooncol, 2006,78:255-260.
34. Cocconi G, Lottici R, Bisagni G, et al. Combination therapy with platinum and etoposide of brain metastases from breast carcinoma. Cancer Invest, 1990,8:327-334.
35. Franciosi V, Cocconi G, Michiara M, et al. Front-line chemotherapy with cisplatin and etoposide for patients with brain metastases from breast carcinoma, nonsmall cell lung carcinoma, or malignant melanoma: a prospective study. Cancer,1999,85:1599-1605.

36. Rivera E, Meyers C, Groves M, et al. Phase I study of capecitabine in combination with temozolomide in the treatment of patients with brain metastases from breast carcinoma. Cancer, 2006, 107:1348-1354.
37. Hedde JP, Neuhaus T, Schuller H, et al. A phase I/II trial of topotecan and radiation therapy for brain metastases in patients with solid tumors. Int J Radiat Oncol Biol Phys, 2007, 68:839-844.
38. Neuhaus T, Ko Y, Muller RP, et al. A phase III trial of topotecan and whole brain radiation therapy for patients with CNS-metastases due to lung cancer. Br J Cancer, 2009, 100:291-297.
39. Lang FF, Chang EL, Abi-Said D. Metastatic brain tumors. In: Winn H, ed. Youman's Neurological Surgery (ed 5th). Philadelphia: Saunders, 2004, 1077-1097.
40. Tsao MN, Lloyd N, Wong R, et al. Whole brain radiotherapy for the treatment of multiple brain metastases. Cochrane Database Syst Rev, 2006, 3:CD003869.